COMPUTED TOMOGRAPHY OF THE

CORONARY
ARTERIES

COMPUTED TOMOGRAPHY OF THE
CORONARY ARTERIES

EDITORS

Pim J de Feyter MD

Gabriel P Krestin MD

CO-EDITORS

Filippo Cademartiri MD

Nico R Mollet MD

Koen Nieman MD

Departments of Cardiology and Radiology
University Hospital Rotterdam
The Netherlands

 Taylor & Francis
Taylor & Francis Group

LONDON AND NEW YORK

A MARTIN DUNITZ BOOK

First published in the United Kingdom in 2005
by Taylor & Francis,
an imprint of the Taylor & Francis Group,
2 Park Square, Milton Park
Abingdon, Oxon OX14 4RN, UK

Tel.:   +44 (0) 1235 828600
Fax.: +44 (0) 1235 829000
Website: www.tandf.co.uk

British Library Cataloguing in Publication Data

Data available on application

Library of Congress Cataloging-in-Publication Data

Data available on application

ISBN 1-84184-439-X

Distributed in North and South America by

Taylor & Francis
2000 NW Corporate Blvd
Boca Raton, FL 33431, USA

Within Continental USA
Tel.: 800 272 7737; Fax.: 800 374 3401
Outside Continental USA
Tel.: 561 994 0555; Fax.: 561 361 6018
E-mail: orders@crcpress.com

Distributed in the rest of the world by
Thomson Publishing Services
Cheriton House
North Way
Andover, Hampshire SP10 5BE, UK
Tel.: +44 (0) 1264 332424
E-mail: salesorder.tandf@thomsonpublishingservices.co.uk

Composition by Parthenon Publishing
Printed and bound by T. G. Hostench S.A., Spain

Contents

Preface

Fast electron-beam computed tomography (CT) was first introduced as a tool for non-invasive identification of coronary findings in the early 1990s. Since then, significant advances in X-ray CT technology have occurred, the most notable being the recent introduction of fast spiral CT coronary imaging.

Non-invasive coronary imaging using spiral CT has emerged as a diagnostic tool that permits assessment of the coronary lumen and coronary plaques. We think that reliable non-invasive coronary imaging will revolutionize our current diagnosis and management of asymptomatic high-risk individuals and symptomatic patients with known or unknown coronary artery disease. CT coronary imaging is now already entering a phase of clinical acceptance and the rapid anticipated technical advances foster great hopes that non-invasive CT coronary imaging will become an alternative to conventional diagnostic coronary angiography. A solid understanding of the basic principles of CT is essential for correct clinical application and interpretation of the CT coronary images.

However, many cardiologists and radiologists are not acquainted with CT coronary imaging. This has inspired the compilation of this book: *Computed Tomography of the Coronary Arteries*. It is the culmination of the collaborative efforts of both cardiologists and radiologists who have drawn up a practical CT text explaining the basic principles and applications of CT through the use of numerous illustrations and tables, while at the same time avoiding the complicated technical details of CT imaging. The results of CT coronary imaging would not have been possible without the faithful and friendly cooperation between cardiologists and radiologists in our institution.

We hope this book will serve its goal as a concise, quick reference for the understanding and interpretation of CT coronary imaging.

Pim J de Feyter
Gabriel P Krestin
October 2004

Acknowledgments

The editors wish to express their gratitude to the many individuals employed in both the radiology and cardiology departments of the Erasmus MC, Rotterdam.

Computed Tomography of the Coronary Arteries is a reflection of the efforts of many individuals and without their help this book would not have been possible.

This book would not have become a reality without the much appreciated skilful help of the members of the staff of Taylor & Francis Medical Books, with special thanks to Martin Lister, Karen Kennedy and Hannah Watson.

We would also like to thank Marcel Dijkshoorn, Berend Koudstaal and Ralf Raaijmakers for their assistance in patient preparation, data acquisition and post-processing.

Finally, we would like to thank Denise Vrouenraets for her excellent secretarial assistance, enthusiasm and encouragement.

CHAPTER 1

Basic principles

Cardiac imaging is currently one of the most rapidly advancing fields in clinical cardiology. Continuing technical innovations are expanding the applicability and usefulness of non-invasive imaging modalities such as ultrasound, nuclear imaging, positron emission tomography, magnetic resonance imaging and, most recently, computed tomography (CT). While CT has been an essential imaging tool in general medicine, for a long time it was regarded to be unsuitable for the imaging of fast-moving organs. However, current multislice spiral CT scanners, with rapid gantry rotation, are able to provide detailed and motion-free imaging of the heart and coronary arteries. It is undeniable that spiral CT has entered the arena of non-invasive cardiac imaging, and while its exact role in the clinical setting still needs to be determined, an increase in the number of cardiac spiral CT examinations is anticipated by both cardiologists and radiologists.

COMPUTED TOMOGRAPHY

Computed tomography is one of the many applications of X-ray radiation. The technique was developed in the early 1970s by Godfrey N. Hounsfield, and together with Dr Allan MacLeod Cormack, who contributed mathematical solutions, he received the Nobel Prize in Medicine for his work in 1979. These first computed axial tomography (CAT) scanners required days to scan, and hours to reconstruct a single image of the head. Technical advancement led to faster imaging and reconstruction, whole-body scanners, improved image quality and dynamic imaging protocols. In the interest of cardiovascular imaging, electron-beam CT was developed in the mid-1980s, which is a non-mechanical CT scanner with a high temporal resolution owing to the

absence of rotating parts. In 1990 the first spiral CT scanners, which provided continuous data acquisition while the patient passed through the scanner, were introduced, and in 1998 the first multislice spiral CT scanners appeared, which allowed simultaneous acquisition of several slices per gantry rotation. These high-resolution volumetric scanners resulted in the development of advanced three-dimensional image processing. The significantly shorter scan time of (multislice) spiral CT scanners improved angiographic applications of CT and, because of the accelerated gantry rotation and improved temporal resolution of these latest generation scanners, contrast-enhanced electrocardiogram (ECG) synchronized cardiovascular imaging has become a reality.

COMPUTED TOMOGRAPHY BASICS

The process of CT, which includes CT coronary angiography, involves the following steps: data acquisition, image reconstruction, post-processing, evaluation, reporting and communication (Figure 1.1).

Data acquisition

Data acquisition refers to the collection of X-ray transmission measurements through the patient. It requires an X-ray source which produces a collimated X-ray beam in the shape of a fan. When an X-ray beam passes through an object some of the photons are absorbed or scattered. The reduction of X-ray transmission, which is called attenuation, depends on the atomic composition and density of the traversed tissues and the energy of the photons. After passing through a section of the patient

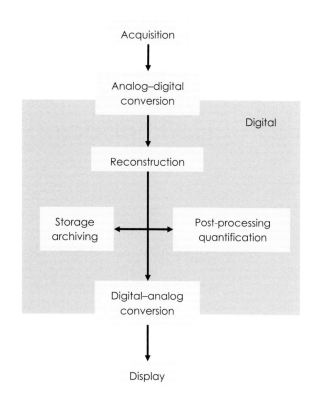

Figure 1.1 Computed tomography procedure

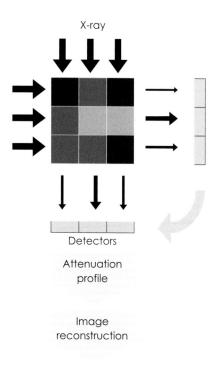

Figure 1.2 Computed tomography data acquisition

the partially attenuated X-rays are collected by X-ray detectors on the opposite side and converted from X-ray photons to electric signals (Figure 1.2). These signals are then converted into digital data, after which the attenuation value is calculated. While the X-ray tube and detectors rotate around the patient, a large number of projections are collected from a large number of angular positions.

Image reconstruction

To create images from the X-ray measurements reconstruction algorithms, including a sequence of reconstruction procedures, should be followed (Figure 1.3). Today, most scanners apply an algorithm called filtered back-projection or convolution method. First the measured X-rays are pre-processed, which is necessary to correct for beam hardening and scattered radiation. After pre-processing the raw data are filtered using convolution kernels. Either smooth or sharp images can be reconstructed based on the selected kernel type. Because the patient moves through the gantry during the scan, the X-ray measurements are acquired at different longitudinal positions. To reconstruct a slice at a certain longitudinal position, the attenuation measurements of at least 180° of the X-ray tube rotation are required. By interpolation of measurements adjacent to the plane position, and weighted according to the respective distance of the measurements to that plane position, a complete set of raw data is created (Figure 1.4). A back-projection technique is then used to calculate the density values within the plane from the filtered and interpolated X-ray measurements. In non-ECG-gated CT scans projections from a full 360° rotation are used. To improve the temporal resolution only half of the projections are used for cardiac scanning, assuming that each 180° rotation of projections is complementary to the other. The consequence of the partial scan algorithm is a decreased signal-to-noise level.

Image processing

The digital axial source images can be converted to electrical signals and displayed on screen using a gray scale, but in the case of cardiovascular CT some post-processing will often be performed prior to evaluation. In order to do so the data are transferred to a computer with

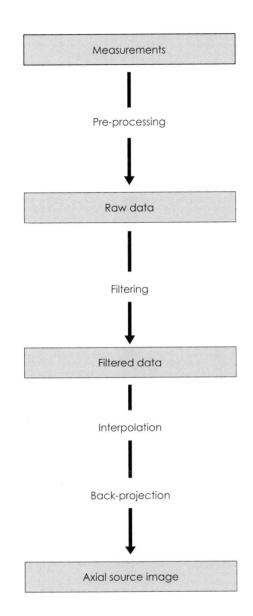

Figure 1.3 Computed tomography image reconstruction

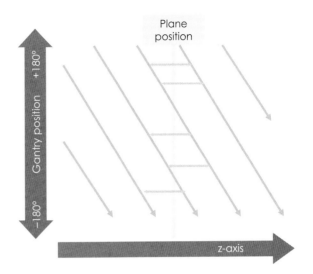

Figure 1.4 Interpolation of the spiral data. Because the table moves continuously, all projections are acquired at slightly different table positions. By a weighted interpolation of the measurements adjacent to the plane position, a complete set of measurements is created and an image can be reconstructed using back-projection algorithms

reconstructions containing more than 200 slices each, will require at least 500 MB. Data can be archived on various magnetic and optical media. Alternatively, digital archiving using a PACS system may be preferred for convenient exchange and retrieval of data. To assure communication of imaging data between various imaging modalities, digital archives, evaluation workstations, printers, etc. from different manufacturers, a standard called DICOM (Digital Imaging and Communication in Medicine) has been developed.

Image display

Contrary to continuous analog images, CT images are digital or numerical images. The attenuated X-ray that reaches the detector is transformed into an analog electrical signal and then converted into a discrete digital format that can be processed by computer. The CT images on screen are an analog visual representation of binary images that have been digitally processed.

The image consists of a matrix of discrete density values that are the result of sampling and computer processing (Figure 1.5). The display of these binary data on the screen can be influenced by a number of factors. The

post-processing and/or quantification software. After (three-dimensional) data manipulation the results can be shown on screen or printed on film or paper.

Data storage

Data can be stored on film but, particularly if additional post-processing is anticipated in the future, digital storage is preferable. A single CT slice is approximately 500 kB. A complete cardiac study, including several

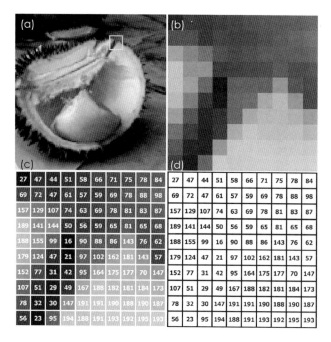

Figure 1.5 Digitization. Detail of a (high-resolution) digitization of a photographed durian fruit (a). The measurements of a detail of the sampled original (analog) image (b) can be displayed within a numerical matrix, but are better interpreted using gray scale (c) and (d)

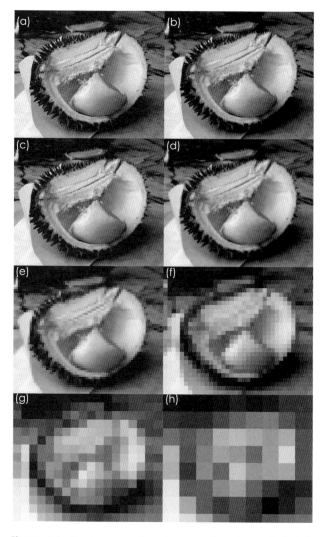

Figure 1.6 Image resolution. Image of a durian fruit (a), which will be considered as a continuous image, can be digitized by sampling and quantifying the (average) density at a specified number of locations. As the matrix size and the number of samples decreases (from (b) to (h)), partial voluming will increase and image detail will be lost

size of the matrix is related to the detail that can be observed (Figure 1.6). When the matrix size is fixed, the spatial resolution can be improved by decreasing the area that is displayed, i.e. by reducing the field-of-view (Figure 1.7). If the matrix size is 512×512 elements and the field-of-view is 25×25 cm, then the size of the pixels or image elements is 0.5×0.5 mm. If the fundamental sampling resolution is sufficient, then the spatial resolution can be increased to $0.2 \times 0.2\,mm^2$ by reducing the field-of-view to $10 \times 10\,cm^2$.

The CT density values are expressed in Hounsfield units (HU) and the density value range is from −1024 to +3071 HU. Theoretically this entire range could be displayed in a gradually sliding scale from black to white according to the CT density values. Unfortunately the human eye is incapable of distinguishing these fine nuances. Therefore, it is important to adjust the display setting in such a way that the range of density values of tissues or structures to be examined are displayed with optimal contrast (Figure 1.8). The window level indicates which density value is in the middle of the displayed gray scale, and determines which attenuation levels or tissue types are visualized. The window width indicates which density values around the window level

are within the gray scale display. Therefore, the width determines the image contrast (Figure 1.9). All matrix elements with density values beyond the window limits appear as either white or black on the screen.

The density value of water is predefined at 0 HU. The density value of soft tissues, such as non-enhanced muscle and blood, vary between approximately −100 HU and +200 HU, while fat tissue is at the lower end of that scale and bone or other calcified tissues have higher-density values. Using routine intravenous contrast-enhancement protocols and materials, the density value of the arterial blood is increased to a level between

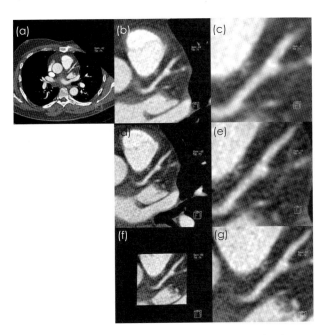

Figure 1.7 Field of view. At a given matrix size the image quality can be improved by decreasing the field of view in the original reconstruction. In the first series the entire thorax is reconstructed and a section of the left anterior descending coronary artery is magnified (a)–(c). In the second series a section of approximately 10×10cm is reconstructed and magnified (d) and (e). In the third series only the proximal left anterior descending (LAD) artery is reconstructed providing superior image resolution compared to the previous magnifications (f) and (g)

+200 HU and +400 HU. Metal has density values that overlap and exceed bone. Air and lung tissue have very low-density values (Figure 1.10).

Taking these values into consideration, the window level of a contrast-enhanced CT image is set at around +250 HU and the window width at 400 HU. This allows appreciation of the contrast-enhanced blood and its relation to the surrounding tissues, with the bone structures and other high-density structures displayed as saturated white, and fat and air displayed as saturated black. Depending on the patient, contrast-enhancement and scanning characteristics these settings can be altered to facilitate optimal appreciation of the coronary lumenal integrity.

COMPUTED TOMOGRAPHY DATA ACQUISITION

Sequential CT

From the first CAT scanners until 1990, all CT scanners were sequential scanners that operated by a stop-and-shoot principle. In sequential scanning the table remains immobile at a specific position while one or one set of slices are acquired, after which the table is moved to the

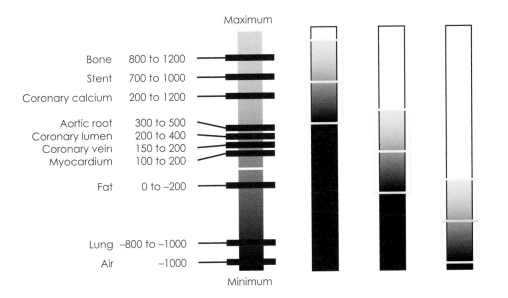

Figure 1.8 Tissue densities and window level and width settings. The tissue attenuation ranges of the various tissues in contrast-enhanced CT angiography are arranged on the first density scale. By setting the window level at a high-density level structures such as bone tissue can be evaluated. An intermediate level around 200 HU allows differentiation of the vessels and their relation to the vessel wall and calcifications. A low window level setting allows appreciation of the lungs. Tissues with density values beyond the boundaries of the window width appear either as saturated white (higher density) or black (lower density)

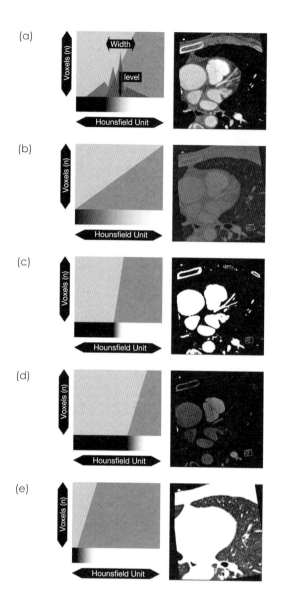

Figure 1.9 Window level and width settings. Display of a digital image can be manipulated by altering the window level and width. The histogram, which represents the number of elements with a specific value within the slice, roughly consists of four tissue types: air and lung tissue, fat tissue, soft tissue and dense tissue (a). The window settings determine how a measured and reconstructed density value is displayed on the screen. To evaluate the coronary arteries the level is set around the density value of the enhanced blood in the coronary arteries (a). Using a wide window all density values are displayed with a slightly different shade (b). Because the human eye is incapable of distinguishing these fine nuances, the structures of interest are not well recognized. Selecting a very narrow width results in sharp images with completely saturated shading of the densities above and below the selected level (c). Increasing the level results in display of high-density structures, i.e. the contrast-enhanced structures and calcified tissue (d), and a low level results in display of the low-density structures, i.e. the lungs (e), and completely saturated display of the other tissues

next position and the acquisition process is repeated (Figure 1.11). Compared with spiral scanning, sequential scanning of non-moving objects is time-inefficient and only limited coverage can be achieved in the same amount of time.

Cardiac sequential CT

Multislice spiral CT scanners are also equipped with a sequential mode for ECG-triggered data acquisition (Figure 1.12). After an R-wave has been registered on the patient's ECG trace the acquisition procedure is initiated and performed during the predicted diastolic phase, based on the duration of the R-to-R intervals of previous cycles. Each time a set of 4–16 slices is acquired, after which the table moves to the next position to wait for the next R-wave. The image quality of triggered multislice CT angiography is regarded to be inferior compared with spiral CT. However, because the radiation is used more efficiently, triggered multislice CT protocols are often preferred for coronary calcium quantification in a preventive setting.

Electron beam CT

Electron beam CT (EBCT) is a non-mechanical sequential CT scanner. Similarly one or more slices are acquired after triggering by the patient's ECG (Figure 1.13). Because of the lack of mechanically rotating parts, the temporal resolution of the scanner is 100 ms, and an acquisition time of 50 ms is available on more recent EBCT scanners. Prospective triggering is applied for both calcium scoring and contrast-enhanced coronary imaging. Either a single acquisition of one (set of) slice(s) or up to three acquisitions can be performed per heart cycle, thus allowing retrospective selection of the most optimal data set.

Spiral CT

In 1990 the first (single slice) spiral CT scanners were introduced. Instead of the stop-and-shoot principle, spiral CT scanners operate with a table that moves at a constant speed and an X-ray-detector system that acquires data continuously (Figure 1.11). As a result, larger sections can be scanned in the same amount of

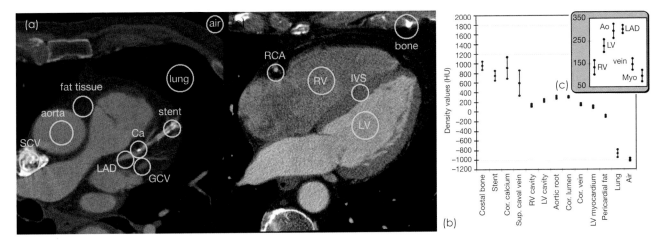

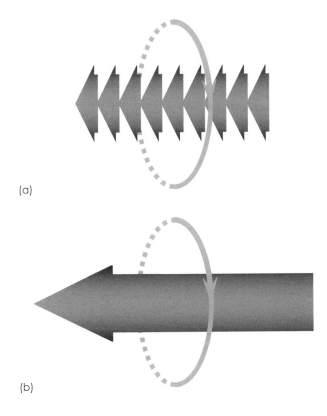

Figure 1.10 Tissue densities. Sampled CT density ranges of tissue within and around the heart. Superior caval vein (SCV), coronary calcium (Ca), great cardiac vein (GCV), right ventricle (RV), left ventricle (LV), interventricular septum (IVS), left anterior descending coronary artery (LAD) and right coronary artery (RCA)

Figure 1.11 Sequential and spiral CT scanning. Sequential scanners acquire one (set of) slices, after which the table is advanced to the next plane position (a). Spiral scanners acquire data continuously while the table moves at a constant speed (b)

time. Particularly vascular CT, which requires dynamic contrast enhancement, benefited from this improvement. Although ECG-gated applications of single-slice spiral CT scanners were explored, insufficient spatial and temporal resolution and a long scan time prevented detailed evaluation of the coronary arteries.

Continuous movement of the couch and continuous scanning have a number of consequences for the scanner hardware. Originally, cables physically connected the rotating and stationary scanner parts, which made continuous rotation impossible. Spiral CT scanners use slip-ring technology to allow continuous rotation of the tube without cable wrap-around. Essentially, energy and scan data are transmitted between the rotating and stationary scanner parts via electrically conductive brushes and rotating rings. Because the X-ray tube generates energy for an extended period a better heat storage capacity is required. Also, the large amount of data that is being produced in a very short period needs storage and processing.

Multislice CT

Instead of a single-detector row, multislice spiral CT scanners have several parallel detector rows, which allow simultaneous acquisition of several slices (Figures 1.14 and 1.15). As a result larger sections can be scanned in a shorter time. This is particularly useful for cardiac

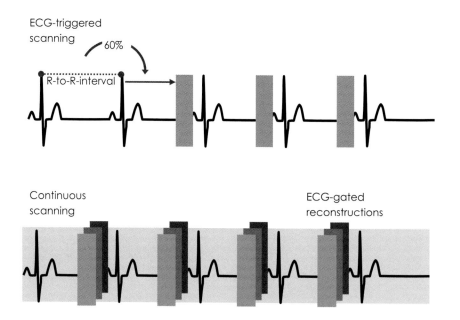

Figure 1.12 Electrocardiogram (ECG)-synchronized image reconstruction. Sequential scan protocols use prospective ECG triggering to synchronize the data acquisition to the motion of the heart. Based on the measured duration of previous heart cycles, the scan of one or more slices is initiated at a pre-specified moment after the R-wave, for instance at 60% of the previous R-to-R intervals. Spiral CT scanners acquire data continuously and record the patient's ECG during the scan. Isocardiophasic images are reconstructed using retrospective ECG gating. The reconstruction window can be positioned anywhere within the R-to-R interval, and images can be created during any phase

acquisitions which deal with an inherently longer scan time compared to organs without movement.

Cardiac spiral CT

To image the heart and particularly the coronary arteries the requirements for a CT scanner are more demanding than those for non-moving organs. To freeze cardiac motion the temporal resolution needs to be high, which requires a rapid rotation speed. The spatial resolution must be adequate to image the small coronary arteries, which requires thin detectors. The entire acquisition needs to be performed during a single breath hold, which requires a short scan time.

In 1998 four-slice spiral CT scanners were introduced with a rotation time of 500 ms and a collimated detector width varying from 0.5 to 1.25 mm, depending on the manufacturer and scan protocol. Using partial scan reconstruction algorithms the reconstruction time was reduced to approximately 250 ms, which proved sufficient to visualize the coronary arteries without motion artifacts during the diastolic phase.

In 2002 16-slice spiral CT scanners were first used for coronary imaging. The rotation time of some of these scanners is now less than 400 ms, the slice thickness varies between 0.5 and 0.75 mm, and a complete scan can be performed in less than 20 s.

ECG-gated image reconstruction

Imaging of the heart requires acquisition or image reconstruction that is synchronized to the motion of the heart (Figure 1.12). Sequential CT scanners, including EBCT, acquire slices prospectively triggered by the patient's ECG. Spiral CT scanners acquire continuous overlapping data throughout the cardiac cycle. Afterwards the recorded ECG is used to select spiral data that have been acquired during the same cardiac phase to reconstruct slices. Because the data have been acquired continuously, reconstruction of any cardiac phase can be performed. To reduce radiation exposure the X-ray tube can be modulated prospectively. Guided by the ECG the output is decreased during the systolic cardiac phase, while full output occurs during an inter-

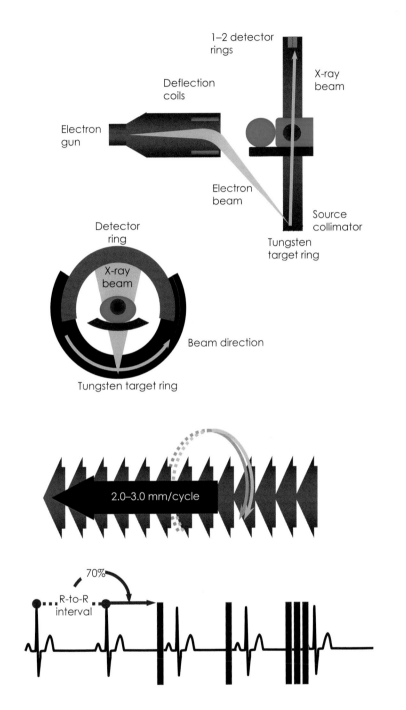

Figure 1.13 Electron beam computed tomography (EBCT) data acquisition. An electron beam is generated and directed along a tungsten ring in the gantry below the patient couch. As the electrons hit the target ring, X-rays are created and a narrow fan beam is passed through the patient after collimation. One or more detector rings are positioned on the opposite side of the gantry to collect the attenuated radiation. After each image acquisition the patient couch is advanced 2–3mm to the next position to perform the next scan. Newer types of EBCT can acquire between one and three or one set of images per heart cycle

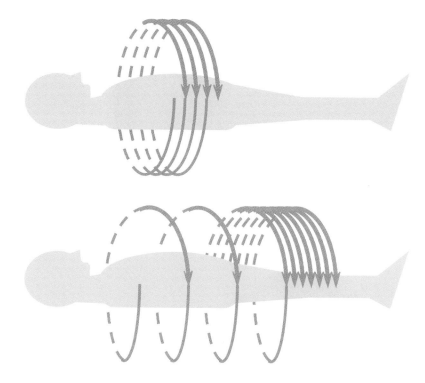

Figure 1.14 Single and multislice spiral CT scanning. Instead of only one detector row, multislice spiral CT scanners are equipped with multiple detector rows which allow for simultaneous acquisition of a number of slices. As a result data can be acquired faster, or longer sections can be scanned in the same amount of time

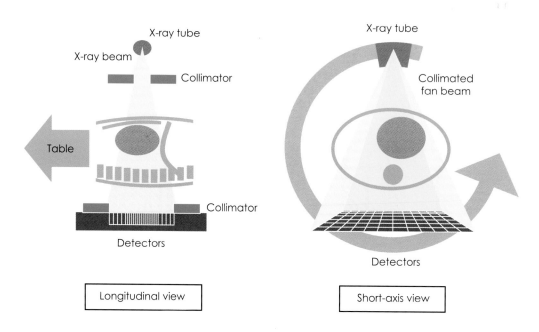

Figure 1.15 Multislice spiral CT. The X-ray tube and the detectors rotate in an opposing position of the gantry around the patient. During continuous X-ray emission a collimated roentgen beam is passed through the patient and the attenuated radiation is collected while the patient on the couch is advanced continuously through the gantry. Instead of one detector row, several parallel detector rows acquire data, which allows accelerated scanning and a short scan time

val within the diastolic phase that is long enough to allow reconstruction of slightly different phases within the diastolic phase. In this way the total radiation exposure can be reduced by 30–40% depending on the heart rate of the patient. The advantages and disadvantages of triggered versus gated image acquisition and reconstruction are presented in Table 1.1.

IMAGE QUALITY AND CHARACTERISTICS (Table 1.2)

Temporal resolution

While the temporal resolution is of little importance when imaging non-moving organs, it is crucial in cardiac imaging[1,2]. The temporal resolution is defined as the required time for data acquisition per slice. In terms of cardiac spiral CT, it refers to the length of the reconstruction window during each heart cycle. It is comparable to the shutter time of a photo camera, and should ideally be infinitely short in order to avoid motion artifacts on the image. Displacements of the object during data acquisition cause streak artifacts that originate from the inability of the reconstruction algorithm to deal with the voxel attenuation inconsistency. The temporal resolution is influenced by scanner characteristics such as the rotation time, as well as the reconstruction algorithm. At a fixed exposure time, the relative temporal resolution can be improved by slowing down the moving object. In case of cardiac imaging this means reducing the heart rate with beta-blockers. Motion that is not related to the cardiac contraction includes swallowing and respiratory motion, which can also cause similar artifacts (Figure 1.16).

Spatial resolution

The spatial resolution refers to the degree of blurring in the image and the ability to discriminate objects and structures of small size. It depends on geometric factors of the CT equipment and factors related to the image reconstruction. Some of the scanner-related factors that cannot be influenced are focal spot size, detector size and the distance between these two. Ideally, both the focal spot and detector size would be infinitely small. Additionally, the resolution improves with the number of acquired projections per rotation. The selected colli-

mation and detector width, as well as the slice thickness, are to a certain degree operator-dependent. When the spatial resolution is insufficient compared to the size of the objects that are being examined, partial voluming will occur (Figure 1.17). This means that a weighted average of the various tissue densities within the image element is displayed. Factors related to the image reconstruction include filtering, the size of the area that is

Table 1.1 Triggered versus gated image acquisition and reconstruction

ECG synchronization	Prospective triggering	Retrospective gating
Reconstruction of multiple cardiac phases	–	+
Multisegmental reconstruction algorithms	–	+
Radiation exposure	+	+++
Vulnerability to arrhythmia	++	+
Retrospective ECG editing	–	+
Slice thickness compared to detector width	=	>
Overlapping slice reconstruction	–	+

ECG, electrocardiogram

Table 1.2 Image quality parameters

Predefined
Rotation time
Detector width
Number of detectors
Patient size
Arrhythmia and heart rate

Operator dependent
Tube current
Tube voltage
Detector collimation
Pitch
Scan range
Contrast enhancement
Heart rate

Reconstruction
Kernel
Reconstruction increment
Field of view
ECG synchronization

ECG, electrocardiogram

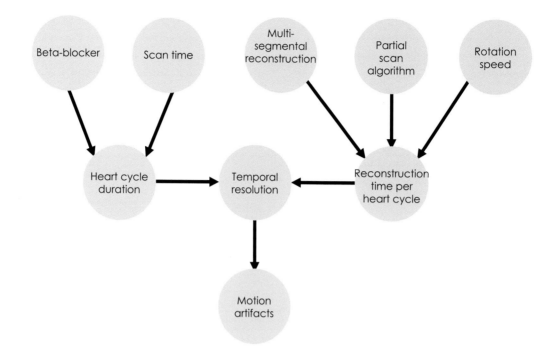

Figure 1.16 Temporal resolution. Factors that influence the (relative) temporal resolution of multislice CT

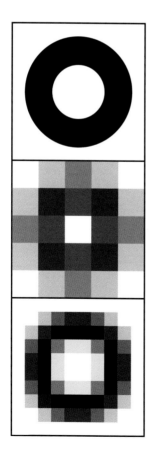

Figure 1.17 Partial voluming. When one image element, a pixel or voxel, contains more than one type of tissue, the density value of the image element will represent a weighted average of both. When a black ring on a white background is digitized, the image consists of various shades of gray depending on the amount of black and white that is sampled within the pixel. While, with a lower resolution none of the pixels contain only a 'black ring', at a higher resolution a number of pixels contain the maximum density without partial voluming. Although the ring becomes easier to recognize, partial voluming or volume averaging will be present around the edges, regardless of the matrix size or spatial resolution

reconstructed, and the size of the image matrix (Figures 1.6 and 1.7).

Contrast resolution

The degree of contrast to differentiate between tissues with varying attenuation characteristics is called the contrast resolution. Because CT has a much better contrast resolution than conventional radiography, tissues with only very small differences in density can be distinguished. The contrast resolution is affected by a number of fixed factors such as the detector sensitivity and the patient size. Factors that can be influenced include the radiation intensity (the current and voltage of the X-ray tube), the slice thickness, reconstruction filtering and image noise (Figure 1.18). Additionally, the display of the tissue contrast is affected by the window settings. The display size and the distance of the radiographer from the screen influence the perception of contrast resolution. Image noise, which is the fluctuation of the measurement compared to the nominal density, negatively affects the contrast resolution. The amount of noise is related to a number of the above-mentioned factors, including the radiation intensity, the slice thickness and detector size.

High-density artifacts and beam hardening

Apart from motion-related streak artifacts and partial voluming related to the spatial resolution, which are discussed above, image degradation can be caused by high-density material and beam-hardening artifacts. Star-shaped metal or high-density artifacts are created when radiation is completely absorbed by high-density objects. In case of cardiac imaging these objects include pacemaker wires, prosthetic valves, surgical clips, indicators at the anastomosis site of bypass grafts, sternal wires and stents (Figure 1.19). Influx of high-density contrast also causes a combination of motion and high-density artifacts. High-density artifacts also play a role in bone structures. Whether subtle high-density artifacts are caused by calcium deposits in the coronary vessel wall and thereby affect the evaluation of coronary arteries is uncertain.

While the heterochromatic X-ray beam passes through the body, the photon spectrum changes. An unequal absorption of low-energy photons results in a shift of the average energy level to the high-energy photons. Because these high-energy photons are less absorbed this causes so-called beam-hardening artifacts.

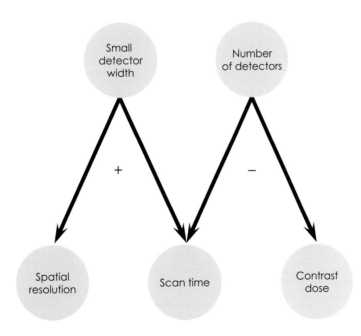

Figure 1.18 Interaction between the number of detectors, the detector width, the spatial resolution and the scan time

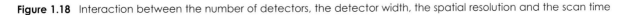

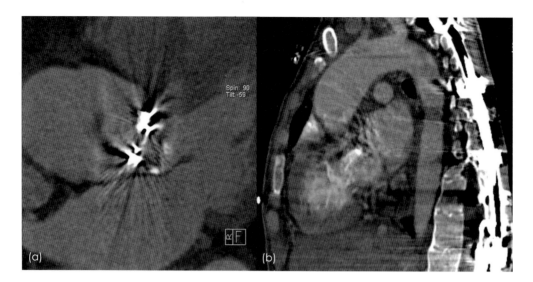

Figure 1.19 Metal artifacts. Artifacts caused by a prosthetic valve (a) and by metal supporting the spine (b)

SCANNING PARAMETERS

The relevant predefined and operator-defined scanning parameters involved with cardiac CT are discussed below.

Tube voltage

The current of the X-ray tube determines the energy of the X-ray radiation, or the hardness of the X-ray. Using a high current (kV), a lower portion of the radiation will be absorbed. A high tube voltage will improve the image contrast (Figure 1.20).

Tube current

The tube current determines the quantity of X-ray radiation, or the number of photons. Using a high tube current results in a higher sampling rate and decreases image noise. A high tube current improves the image quality, but also increases the total radiation exposure (Figure 1.20).

Rotation time

The rotation time of the system is an important parameter for cardiac CT scanning. The rotation time is usu-
ally fixed, and should be as short as possible to reduce motion artifacts. Currently multislice spiral CT scanners have a rotation time that varies between 0.38 and 0.60 s. To reconstruct an axial slice, projections from a half gantry rotation are required. When data from a single rotation are used to synthesize an image, the temporal resolution is equal to half of the gantry rotation time (Figure 1.21).

If the same object section is scanned twice (by different detectors) during the same phase of two consecutive cardiac cycles, it will be possible to combine these data, thereby reducing the effective spatial resolution. If the heart rate in relation to the gantry rotation is optimal, two non-overlapping 90° rotations during the same contraction phase of consecutive heart cycles can be used for image reconstruction, effectively resulting in a temporal resolution of a quarter of the rotation time. However, if for example the rotation rate is exactly twice as high as the heart rate, then the isophasic data of consecutive heart cycles are not complementary, and no improvement of the effective temporal resolution is possible. Therefore, using bisegmental or biphasic reconstruction algorithms results in a temporal resolution between a quarter and a half of the rotation time, varying with the heart rate in relation to the scanner rotation time. Reconstruction algorithms that combine data from three or four cycles are available with a potential temporal resolution between an eighth and a half of the rotation time (Figure 1.22). These algorithms are most optimal when the heart rate is constant, the ECG signal

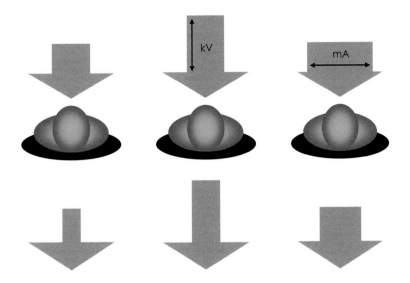

Figure 1.20 Tube current and voltage. Increasing the tube voltage and the energy of the radiation (represented by the length of the arrow) will result in reduced attenuation. Alternatively, a larger quantity of roentgen can be emitted to increase the number of photons that reach the detectors (represented by the width of the arrow), which also improves the quality of the images

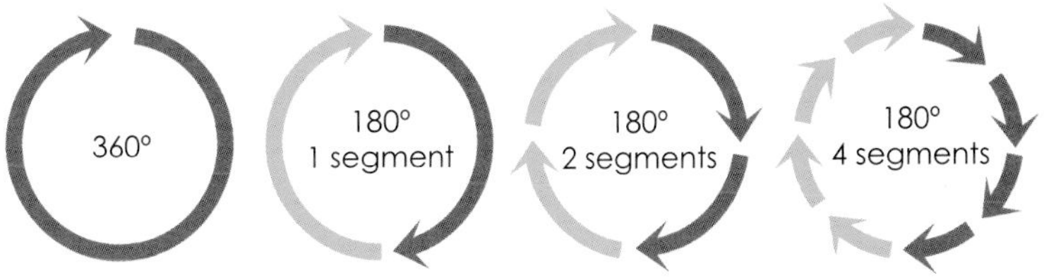

	360°	180° 1 segment	180° 2 segments	180° 4 segments
Effective temporal resolution (relative to rotation time (T))	T	0.5T	0.25–0.5T	0.125–0.5T
Effective temporal resolution (in ms at 420 ms rotation time)	420	210	105–210	52.5–210
Minimal sampling rate (cycles/position)	1×	1×	2×	4×

Figure 1.21 Reconstruction algorithms in cardiac multislice CT. In non-cardiac imaging data from an entire rotation are used for image reconstruction. For cardiac scanning a partial scan is used for image reconstruction. By combining data acquired at the same position during the same phase of two or four cardiac cycles, the effective temporal resolution can be reduced. Depending on the actual heart rate during acquisition and the rotation time of the scanner the effective temporal resolution varies between 50% and 25% (two segments) or 12.5% (four segments), of the rotation time of the scanner. Using these multi-segmental reconstruction algorithms requires multiple sampling of the same position, with a shorter scan range and increased radiation exposure

is reliable and no arrhythmia occurs, since they rely on an identical contraction pattern with time-consistent positioning of the cardiac structures during each consecutive heart cycle. Furthermore, multisegmental reconstruction of slices requires multiple sampling of the same section during a number of cardiac cycles. If the heart rate of the patient is low, this will require slower table advancement (see next section on pitch).

Table advancement and pitch

The pitch is the table advancement per rotation divided by the width of the collimated detector width. To scan non-moving body sections the table advancement should be as high as possible while ensuring sufficient data acquisition. For non-gated scan protocols, the pitch usually varies between one and two. A pitch of one results in optimal image quality but can be increased to shorten the scan time (Figure 1.23). With a higher pitch the scan time will be shorter and the radiation exposure less, while the effective slice thickness will increase. For cardiac scanning, each position needs to be sampled during at least one entire heart cycle; therefore, the pitch is lower, far less than the width of the collimated detectors. Optimally, the pitch should be variable, and increase with the heart rate of the patient. If multisegmental reconstruction algorithms are used the pitch needs to be sufficiently low to ensure sampling of each position during several cycles.

Patients with fast heart rates

The reliability of multislice CT (MSCT) coronary angiography is better in patients with a low heart rate[1,2]. In patients with a heart rate below 60–65 beats/min adequate image quality to assess qualitatively lumenal narrowing is possible in the proximal branches and in most of the smaller branches and side branches (Figure 1.24). Unfortunately, the majority of patients have a resting heart rate above 65 beats/min, particularly prior to a medical examination. In view of the relatively limited temporal resolution of MSCT, considerable effort has been invested into the development of technology with a faster rotation speed.

Faced with the current limitations there are a number of approaches to improving image quality with respect to motion artifacts in patients with a fast heart rate. By administration of oral or intravenous beta-receptor blocking agents the heart rate can be reduced. The easiest approach is an oral dose of a fast-acting and short-lasting beta-blocker such as metoprolol 1 h before the examination. Alternatively, an intravenous protocol with esmolol can be used. At an increasing infusion rate esmolol is injected resulting in an immediate and short-lasting heart rate deceleration. While the eventual heart rate with oral beta-blocking is unpredictable, intravenous esmolol can be administered until the desired heart rate has been achieved. Because of the short-lasting effect, this protocol needs to be executed in the CT suite and may take some time, during which the scanner is not being used. When the use of beta-blockers is considered, the absence of contraindications and possible side-effects should be known with certainty. In case of an atrioventricular conduction delay, heart failure or low blood pressure, beta-blockers are contraindicated.

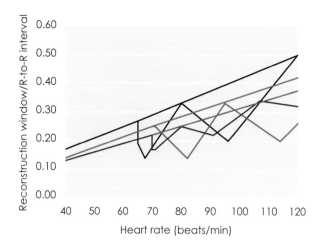

Figure 1.22 The relative temporal resolution, i.e. the ratio of the reconstruction window and the duration of the R-to-R interval, in relation to the patient's heart rate for four-multislice CT (MSCT) scanners with a rotation time of 500 ms, for 16-slice MSCT with a rotation time of 420 ms or 375 ms. The lines between 40 and 65 beats/min show the relative temporal resolution without the use of bisegmental reconstruction algorithms. Multisegmental reconstruction algorithms are generally not used in patients with a low heart rate

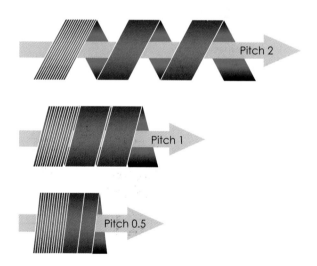

Figure 1.23 Pitch. Using a high pitch the table advancement per gantry rotation is large and extended sections can be scanned in a short period of time. Decreasing the pitch improves the image quality but results in a longer scan time. For cardiac imaging an even smaller pitch of less than one is required, which results in multiple acquisitions of each position to guarantee availability of data during the entire cardiac cycle and allows for multiphasic reconstruction

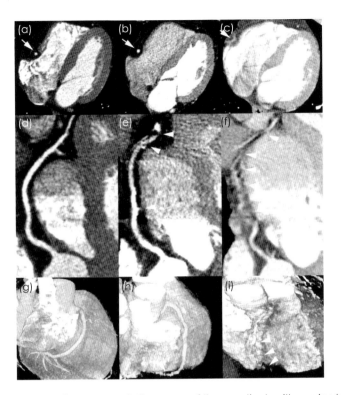

Figure 1.24 Heart rate related image quality. Representative cases of three patients with varying heart rates. The right coronary artery is displayed at a heart rate of 49 beats/min, 64 beats/min and 81 beats/min (Reproduced with permission from Nieman et al.[2])

Prior to the examination, the patient's resting ECG should be examined and blood pressure measured. During examination the atrioventricular conduction may, in rare cases, be compromised or a symptomatic drop in blood pressure may occur. However, using a low dose of metoprolol, i.e. 100 mg, this rarely occurs. In case of low blood pressure or mild conduction disorders an extended observation period is desirable.

To avoid the use of beta-blockers, and still scan patients with faster heart rates, alternative scanning and reconstruction methods are available (see section on Rotation time). If the heart rate is faster and the pitch remains the same, each position will be scanned during more than one heart cycle. This allows bisegmental or multisegmental reconstruction algorithms to be used that combine data from consecutive acquisitions of the same position during the same cardiac phase, which potentially improves the effective temporal resolution. As previously mentioned, the effectiveness of these algorithms varies with the actual heart rate in relation to the rotation time of the scanner. The effective temporal resolution in relation to the heart rate using different rotation times and multisegment reconstruction algorithms can be found in Figure 1.22. To avoid heart rates with less efficient temporal resolutions some MSCT scanners allow selection of the scanner rotation speed. If a certain heart rate is unfavorable with the fastest rotation speed, a lower rotation speed with a better bisegmental temporal resolution can be selected. This approach requires the heart rate to be stable. Reconstruction algorithms that combine acquisition data from up to four cycles are available but can only be used in very high heart rates without decreasing the table propagation speed. Finally, the use of multisegmental reconstruction algorithms gives the best result when the heart rate is stable. If the R-to-R interval varies data acquired during different heart phases will be combined, resulting in image artifacts.

Scan time

The duration of the scan can be calculated as follows:

$$\text{Scan time} = \frac{\text{scan volume} \times \text{rotation}}{\text{pitch} \times n \times \text{width}}$$

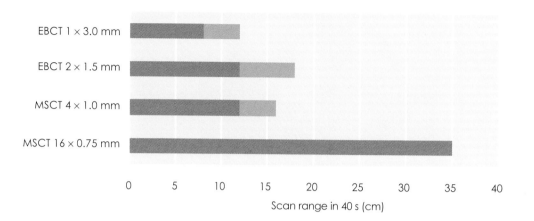

EBCT 1 × 3.0 mm

EBCT 2 × 1.5 mm

MSCT 4 × 1.0 mm

MSCT 16 × 0.75 mm

Scan range in 40 s (cm)

Figure 1.25 Scanner types and scan duration. The time required to scan an average-sized heart, at a heart rate varying from 60 to 90 beats/min, using single-slice electron beam (EB)CT, double-slice EBCT, four-slice multislice (MS)CT and 16-slice MSCT

More and larger detectors (where *n* is the number of detectors), a faster rotation and a higher pitch reduce the scan time of a given scan range.

Because all data are preferably acquired in a single scan, which should be performed while the patient holds his breath and remains completely motionless, the total scan time needs to be as short as possible. ECG-triggered or ECG-gated protocols require a substantially longer scan time (Figure 1.25). Using four-slice MSCT, with a 500-ms rotation time and four 1-mm detector rows the heart can be covered in 35–40 s, which is a considerable period to hold one's breath. In addition to voluntary and involuntary patient movement the long breath-hold time causes acceleration of the heart rate. Using 16-slice technology, with a < 400-ms rotation time and 16×0.75-mm detector rows the scan time is less than 20 s. For comparison, the entire abdominal aorta and femoral run-offs can be scanned using a non-gated protocol and 1.5-mm slices in the same amount of time.

Detector collimation and slice thickness

The collimation describes the number and individual width of the detectors. Most scanners allow selection of a number of different collimations (Figure 1.26). Clearly a thinner collimation results in thinner slices, while selection of a wider detector with thicker collimation increases the scan speed. For coronary imaging the thinnest-slice thickness offers the highest spatial resolution and best diagnostic images (Figure 1.27). A relatively higher radiation dose is, however, required when

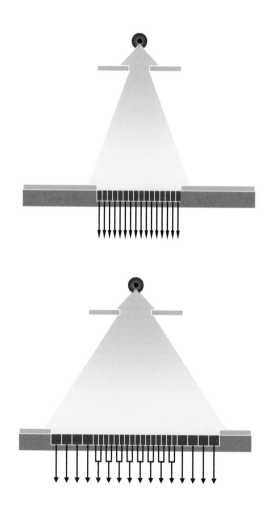

Figure 1.26 Collimation protocols. For high-resolution imaging a detector collimation with the finest-slice thickness is preferable. To increase the longitudinal coverage per second a collimation with thicker slices is selected. Data collected by the thin inner detectors are combined in pairs

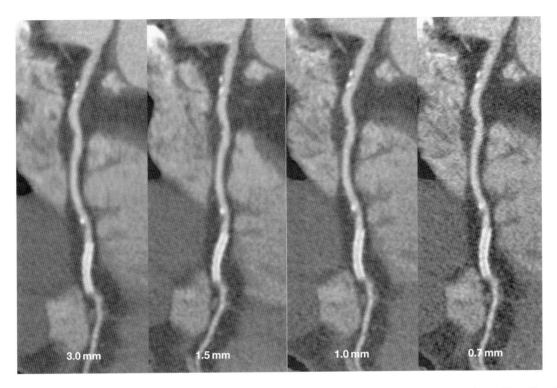

Figure 1.27 Slice thickness. Four reconstructions of the same scan showing a stented right coronary artery with a slice thickness of 3.0, 1.5, 1.0 and 0.7 mm, each with a reconstruction overlap of approximately 50%

using thinner slices to compensate for increased image noise. When sub-millimeter resolution is not essential, a thicker-slice thickness may offer benefits such as better contrast, less radiation exposure, less contrast medium and short scan time.

The *slice sensitivity profile* describes the relation between the detector width and the resultant slice thickness. Because interpolation of the measurements adjacent to the actual slice position is required in spiral scanning protocols, the reconstructed slice is influenced by measurements of structures outside the boundaries of the detector position. This can be visualized by the slice sensitivity profile, which is nearly rectangular for sequential acquisitions. In spiral scanning the effective slice thickness, expressed as the width of the curve at mid-level (full-width-half-maximum) is wider than the detector width, and increases with the pitch (Figure 1.28).

Kernel

The kernel is a modifiable feature that influences the contrast in the images. A soft kernel results in smooth

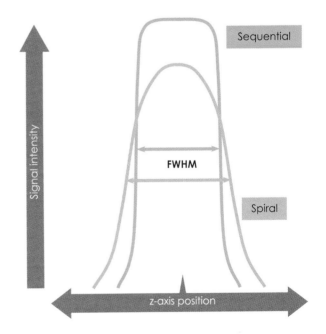

Figure 1.28 Slice sensitivity profile. Due to the interpolation of measurements the effective slice thickness (at full-width-half-maximum (FWHM)) of the reconstructed spiral CT images is slightly increased in comparison to the effective slice thickness of sequentially acquired CT images, at a constant individual detector width

19

images with low image noise, while strong kernels enhance the contrast, improve edge definition but increase the image noise (Figure 1.29). Applying filtering at either end of the spectrum should be avoided, but slight variation may enhance the interpretability of the images. Slightly harder images may improve the image quality in stented vessels and for stenosis quantification, while softer images may be preferable to characterize atherosclerotic plaque composition.

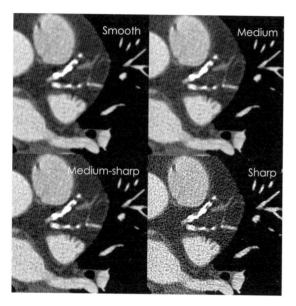

Figure 1.29 Reconstruction kernels. The filtering of the data before reconstruction, showing an axial slice with a severely calcified left coronary artery, can either smooth or sharpen the images, from plane (a) to (d)

Reconstruction increment

Slices with a given thickness can be reconstructed at an overlapping interval, which results in an improved through-plane image quality and a slightly higher (subjective) spatial resolution (Figure 1.30). The high number of overlapping slices improves the quality of three-dimensional reconstructions but increases the processing time and further challenges storage facilities. For coronary angiography an overlap of between 30% and 50% is recommended.

Field of view

While nearly the entire content within the boundaries of the gantry is scanned and available, only the area where the patient or a specific structure is situated is reconstructed. Within this field of view a raster with a predefined number of pixels is reconstructed from the raw data. When coronary imaging is the purpose of the scan, the field of view is placed tightly around the heart to optimize the in-plane spatial resolution. If a specific structure within the heart needs to be examined in detail an additional reconstruction with an even smaller field-of-view can be performed. This is limited by the fundamental spatial resolution of the scanner hardware beyond which further minimization of the field of view is without improvement of the spatial resolution (Figure 1.7).

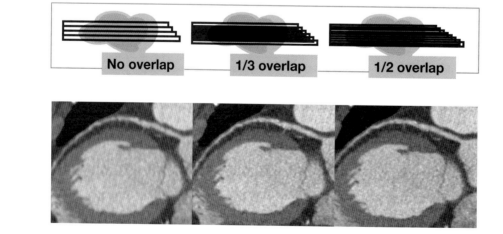

Figure 1.30 Reconstruction increment. Comparison of the longitudinal or through-plane image quality after reconstruction of slices with no, one-third or one-half overlap

ECG synchronization

ECG triggering and ECG gating have been described in detail above. Some matters with respect to the user interference with gating will be discussed here. Reconstruction of images during the exact same cardiac phase requires a good ECG signal. The electrodes should be placed at the appropriate locations on the abdomen and left and right thorax, at locations without electrical interference from the musculature underneath. The gating software interprets the up-slope deviation of the R-wave as t_0. The leads Einthoven I and II will result in the most extreme R-wave deviation in most patients and are therefore best interpreted by the software (Figure 1.31). In patients with conduction disorders or an otherwise unusual ECG configuration, alternative leads should be explored to obtain an ECG signal that is easily analyzed by the scanner. After the acquisition is completed the ECG trace is displayed on screen with indications as to where R-waves were recognized. If an R-wave indication has been misplaced, for instance due to ECG noise, its position can be modified. For coronary imaging the cardiac phase in which coronary displacement is minimal is the mid- to end-diastolic phase. Reconstructions can be performed at time positions relative to the previous or the upcoming R-wave (Figure 1.32). Alternatively a position as a percentage of the R-to-R wave can be selected (Figures 1.33 and 1.34). Which approach is most optimal is a matter of debate and only really matters in case of a heart rate that is not constant. Often a number of reconstructions at slightly varying time positions are compared to determine the most optimal phase. In case of fast or irregular heart rates the end-systolic phase may give the most consistent image quality.

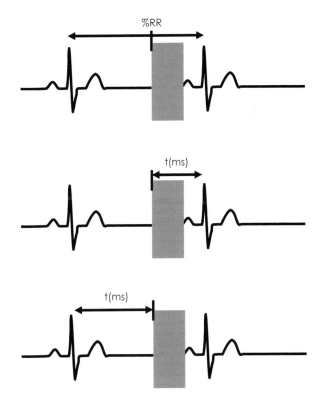

Figure 1.32 Reconstruction window positioning. To ensure consistent isocardiophasic images and avoid interslice discontinuity, reconstruction must take place during the exact same phase within each heart cycle. The scanner's reconstruction software will allow different types of positioning with respect to the ECG. The position can be at a relative position as a percentage of the distance between the consecutive R-waves (RR), or it can be at an absolute time distance (t) with respect to the preceding or upcoming R-wave. There is little consensus about the most optimal method, and particularly in patients with an accelerating or varying heart rate exploration of alternative methods can be worthwhile

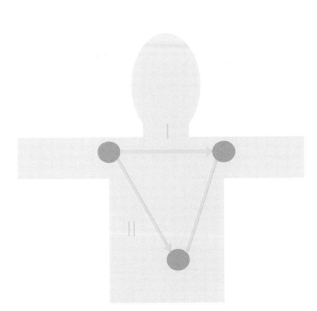

Figure 1.31 Positioning of the electrocardiogram (ECG) leads. The ECG electrodes are usually positioned around the left and right shoulder region at locations that are not affected by disturbing activity from the musculature underneath. The third lead is attached to the lower abdomen. In most patients either an Einthoven I or II configuration will result in a steep and high-amplitude R-wave, which is best interpreted by the scanner

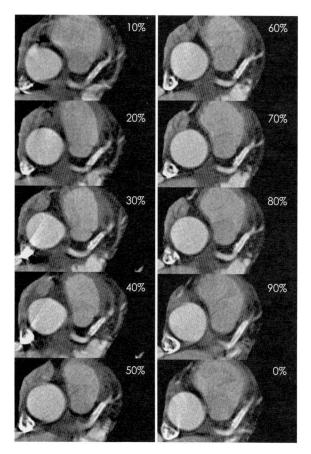

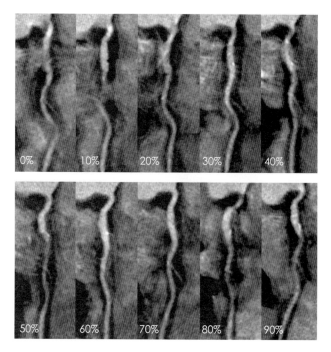

Figure 1.34 Multiphasic reconstruction of an right coronary artery. Ten reconstructions and curved multiplanar reformation of a diseased right coronary artery at different temporal positions within the heart cycle. Reconstruction window positioning is expressed as a percentage of the R-to-R interval

Figure 1.33 Multiphasic reconstruction of a stented LAD. Reconstruction of an axial slice through the left anterior descending artery with a patent stent at ten different temporal positions within the heart cycle. Reconstruction window positioning is expressed as a percentage of the R-to-R interval

LIMITATIONS OF CARDIAC CT

Several limitations and potential pitfalls should be considered when MSCT coronary angiography is performed. They can be related to the technical features and characteristics of MSCT, the examination of a moving organ, interaction of the patient with the acquisition process, and the use of post-processing software. Additionally, quantification of lesions cannot be performed with the same accuracy as compared with conventional coronary angiography.

Limitations related to the CT equipment

MSCT has a spatial resolution, which is fundamentally limited by a number of factors including the quality and width of the detector row and the size of the X-ray tube's focal point. Other factors include the amount of contrast and the size of the field of view. The spatial resolution of the current MSCT scanners has an estimated range of 0.5–0.8 mm in all three dimensions. This means that vessels smaller than 1.0–1.5 mm cannot be evaluated with the same accuracy as larger vessels.

Limitations related to cardiac imaging

Imaging of the heart and coronary arteries is best performed in patients with a slow and stable heart rate. Patients with very irregular heart rates, such as those with atrial fibrillation, should not undergo MSCT coronary angiography, because the end-diastolic volume is different for each consecutive beat and the interslice continuity is poor. In addition, the image reconstruction needs to be performed during the motion-sparse diastolic phase of the heart cycle, and a number of reconstructions may be explored to find the most optimal moment (Figure 1.35). Despite multisegmental reconstruction algorithms, imaging of a patient with an accel-

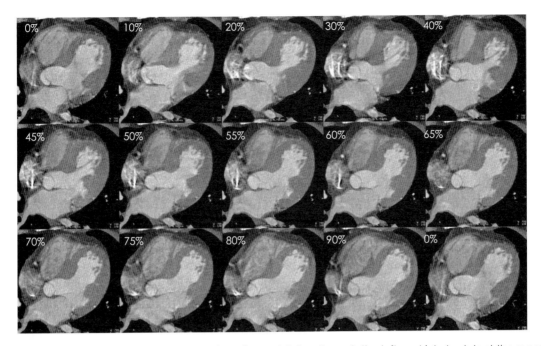

Figure 1.35 Multiphasic reconstruction. Reconstruction of an axial slice through the left ventricle to detect the reconstruction window with the least motion artifact

erated heart rate is less than optimal. Exceptional examples of successful imaging at faster heart rates are often presented as the standard, but in our experience the quality is inconsistent and results in a high number of non-interpretable examinations.

Patient-related aspects

Patients should be completely motionless during the examination. They should feel at ease and be in a comfortable position that can be maintained throughout the procedure. To avoid misinterpretation of the (automatic) instructions, the patient should be briefed in advance and understand the sequence of events, including sensations caused by the contrast material. The scan time should be known to the patient and short enough with respect to the specific patient limitations. Finally, swallowing during the scan should be avoided.

Highly attenuating material, such as calcium and stents, causes beam-hardening artifacts and partial voluming, which can interfere with the interpretation of the lumen diameter. Therefore, the lumen within stents and adjacent to severely calcified vessels are more difficult to evaluate. This will be discussed further in the respective chapters.

Table 1.3 Radiation and influencing factors

Determinants of the total radiation exposure

Scanner parameter
Scanner type
X-ray output (kV and mA)
Pitch
Collimation: slice number and slice width
Scan range
ECG-triggered X-ray tube modulation

Patient characteristics
Gender
Size
Heart rate

RADIATION EXPOSURE (Table 1.3)

MSCT is a roentgen technique and the examination cannot be performed without exposure of the patient to (potentially) harmful radiation. The amount of radiation that the patient is subjected to depends on the scanner type, the scan protocol and patient characteristics. ECG-gated spiral CT requires overlapped scanning to ensure the availability of data from each position during the entire heart cycle. Therefore, the dose is higher than comparable non-gated thoracic protocols. By selecting a higher X-ray tube output the quality of the images will improve, but the radiation dose will increase. Theoretically a detector collimation with thinner slices would not affect the dose. However, because the absolute amount of radiation that reaches the thinner detectors is lower, image noise will increase. To maintain an acceptable contrast-to-noise level the mA settings are often upgraded with thin-detector collimation protocols.

The radiation dose is pitch dependent. When the patient has a fast heart rate the pitch can be increased, while each position is still scanned during an entire cardiac cycle. Because motion artifacts are more frequent in patients with a fast heart rate, multisegmental reconstruction algorithms are applied to improve the effective temporal resolution. This requires sampling of each position during two or more heart cycles, thereby increasing the radiation exposure.

Naturally, the radiation dose depends on the scan range. Because the position of the heart may vary between the overview scan and the actual angiographic data acquisition, there is a tendency to apply safety margins and to avoid missing crucial sections of the heart. With the improved scan speed of the latest multislice spiral CT scanners it is possible to scan an extended range while maintaining an acceptable breath-hold time. It is important to keep in mind that the consequence is an equal increase in radiation.

Radiation-dose terminology (Table 1.4)

From measurements with an ionization chamber the radiation dose of one acquired slice can be calculated using the CT dose index (CTDI) method. The CTDI is equal to the measured-dose distribution divided by the slice width and the number of slices in case of multislice scanners. Because the radiation exposure is higher at the edges of the object the weighted CTDI, or $CTDI_w$, can be calculated as two-thirds of $CTDI_{edge}$ plus one-third $CTDI_{center}$. In case of a volumetric scan, which is usually the case in coronary angiography, the volume $CTDI_w$ can be calculated: $CTDI_{vol} = CTDI_w/pitch$. This is the dose of a single axial slice within a volumetric acquisition, expressed in milligray (mGy). To calculate the dose of an entire scan, or the dose-length product (DLP), the $CTDI_{vol}$ needs to be multiplied by the length of the scan.

The effective dose (E) reflects the potential biological effect of the radiation, which depends on the tissue that is exposed, and is expressed in millisieverts (mSv). It depends on a k value that is specific for the scanned body region. The effective dose is the DLP multiplied by the k value, which is 0.017 for the chest region.

Radiation exposure reduction

There have been a number of publications on the radiation exposure of cardiac CT, some of which were estimations and others actual measurements. Most of the data refer to four-slice spiral CT. Morin and co-workers[3] estimated the effective radiation dose of four-slice MSCT coronary angiography to be between 9.3 and 11.3 mSv. Hunold and colleagues[4] used a phantom to measure the radiation dose during the CT examination, which was calculated to be 6.7–10.9 mSv for men and 8.1–13.0 mSv for women. Phantom experiments with 16-slice MSCT resulted in a radiation dose of 8.1 mSv (men) and 10.9 mSv (women)[5]. As mentioned before, the actual radiation dose is further influenced by the scan parameters used.

Table 1.4 Radiation-dose terminology

	Meaning	Calculation
CT dose index (CTDI)	radiation dose of a single slice	
Weighted CTDI ($CTDI_w$)	dose corrected for the inhomogeneous attenuation	$^2/_3 CTDI_{edge} + {}^1/_3 CTDI_{center}$
Volume CTDI ($CTDI_{vol}$)	slice dose in a scan with multiple acquisitions	$CTDI_w/pitch$
Dose-length product (DLP)	total dose of a scan with multiple acquisitions	$CTDI_{vol} \times length$
Effective dose (R)	biological effect (region dependent) of an acquisition	$DLP \times k$

k is 0.017 for chest region

In comparison, the effective radiation dose of a non-gated thoracic CT angiogram varies between 5 and 7 mSv. The exposure during conventional angiography varies and is dependent on the indication for the examination, the equipment used and the angiographer. The radiation dose during a routine angiographic procedure varies between approximately 3 and 10 mSv. Therefore, radiation dose considerations are not in favor of MSCT. The yearly exposure from natural sources is approximately 3.6 mSv. Finally, the dose of an angiographic EBCT examination using 3.0-mm slices varies between 1.1 and 2.0 mSv[3,4]. The exposure is lower because radiation is only applied during a short period within the heart cycle when data acquisition takes place. More recent EBCT scanners acquire more than one slice per heart cycle with a reduced detector width, which will increase the total radiation dose to maintain acceptable signal-to-noise.

The purpose of coronary CT will depend on the eventual radiation exposure and possible consequences of exposure. While a higher dose is acceptable when CT is used as an alternative to other X-ray techniques, such as conventional catheter-based angiography, the radiation dose should be significantly reduced if MSCT were to be used at an earlier stage of coronary artery disease or as a screening tool. Therefore, manufacturers are investing considerable effort in order to reduce the radiation dose. One approach involves alternation of the X-ray tube output during the examination (Figure 1.36). Although scanning is performed throughout the cardiac cycle, only data acquired during the diastolic phase are generally used for coronary evaluation. By lowering the output during systole by means of prospective ECG triggering, while maintaining a nominal output during diastole, the total exposure can be reduced without compromising the image quality. ECG-triggered X-ray tube modulation decreased the estimated radiation dose of four-slice MSCT calcium scoring from 2.0 mSv (men) and 2.5 mSv (women), to 1.0 mSv and 1.4 mSv, respectively[6]. With 16-slice MSCT the exposure could be reduced from nearly 10 mSv to 4.3 mSv, using tube modulation for coronary imaging[5].

Another approach involves X-ray tube output modulation depending on the X-ray tube in relation to the patient. Because the amount of tissue that needs to be traversed is considerably more in a lateral direction compared to a frontal direction, a lower exposure is sufficient for adequate image quality in the latter direction.

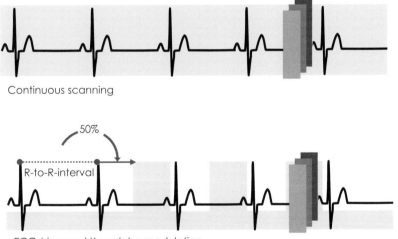

Continuous scanning

50%

R-to-R-interval

ECG-triggered X-ray tube modulation

Figure 1.36 X-ray tube output modulation. While standard scan protocols require continuous output of the X-ray tube, more advanced protocols allow alternation of the output throughout the data acquisition procedure. Prospectively triggered by the ECG, the output of the roentgen tube is decreased during the systolic phase, when coronary evaluation is rarely performed, while nominal exposure is generated during the diastolic phase to ensure optimal image quality. The period of full exposure should be long enough for subtle variation of the reconstruction window position and the possibility to select the most optimal phase. Ideally, exposure during systole is sufficient for functional assessment of the ventricular performance. The exposure reduction is highest when the heart rate is low (at a constant scan pitch). Additionally, this application requires an ECG signal that is free of noise or artifacts, as incorrect ECG signal reading can result in inadequate exposure during the diastolic phase, which in contrast to the positioning of the reconstruction window, cannot be edited after the acquisition of data

REFERENCES

1. Giesler T, Baum U, Ropers D, et al. Noninvasive visualization of coronary arteries using contrast-enhanced multidetector CT: influence of heart rate on image quality and stenosis detection. Am J Roentgenol 2002; 179: 911–16

2. Nieman K, Rensing BJ, van Geuns RJ, et al. Non-invasive coronary angiography with multislice spiral computed tomography: impact of heart rate. Heart 2002; 88: 470–4

3. Morin RL, Gerber TC, McCollough CH. Radiation dose in computed tomography of the heart. Circulation 2003; 107: 917–22

4. Hunold P, Vogt FM, Schmermund A, et al. Radiation exposure during cardiac CT: effective doses at multidetector row CT and electron-beam CT. Radiology 2003; 226: 145–52

5. Jakobs TF, Becker CR, Ohnesorge B, et al. Multislice helical CT of the heart with retrospective ECG gating: reduction of radiation exposure by ECG-controlled tube current modulation. Eur Radiol 2002; 12: 1081–6

6. Trabold T, Buchgeister M, Kuttner A, et al. Estimation of radiation exposure in 16-detector row computed tomography of the heart with retrospective ECG-gating. Rofo Fortschr Geb Rontgenstr Neuen Bildgeb Verfahr 2003; 175: 1051–5

CHAPTER 2

Image post-processing

Image post-processing is defined as the process of using imaging techniques to modify the initial axial images (the source images) to make them more useful to the observer[1,2]. Post-processing is useful because it allows clinically relevant information to be extracted from the enormous amount of data (more than 300–800 axial images) that is generated by a multislice CT (MSCT) acquisition from a single thoracic examination. The use of these post-processing techniques allows the investigators to understand better the complex coronary artery anatomy and related coronary abnormalities, which can be extremely difficult to ascertain from the large number of axial images. The usefulness and quality of image post-processing is highly related to the in-plane and through-plane resolution of MSCT. The data that form the CT slice are sectioned into elements, the width indicated on the x-axis and the height on the y-axis (Figure 2.1a), to create a two-dimensional square indicated as a pixel (picture element). However, there is a third component, the thickness of the slice, which is indicated on the z-axis. Taking the thickness into account turns the square (pixel) into a cube which is referred to as a voxel (volume element) (Figure 2.1b). The thickness of the slice is important, because the X-ray beam passes only through the selected slice thickness, thereby eliminating superimposition and radiation scatter of adjacent structures, which creates high-quality images. In computerized imaging, pictures are composed of pixels. The region of interest is mathematically divided into voxels. In each voxel the signals are averaged and turned into a number, which eventually represents a certain level on the gray scale. These numbers are used to create a picture consisting of pixels. The pixels are arranged in an image matrix, which is a grid consisting of rows (x-axis) and columns (y-axis). The matrix size used for CT is generally 512×512 pixels. The field of view (FOV) is

the diameter of the area being imaged. The pixel size is determined by the ratio of the FOV and matrix or:

$$\text{Pixel size} = \frac{\text{FOV}}{\text{Matrix size}}$$

The smaller is the pixel (or voxel) the higher is the resolution.

The voxel is the fundamental unit of the volume. Adding up all the voxels of the volume and applying a post-processing algorithm such as volume rendering will result in the anatomical representation of the data set. In terms of image quality, the smaller is the voxel the better is the spatial resolution of the image (Figure 2.1c). It is important to note that the shape of voxels may differ and, depending on the slice thickness, the voxel may be constructed as an isotropic voxel, i.e. x-y-z measurements are identical, or as an anisotropic voxel, i.e. x-y are similar but z is usually larger.

Isotropic imaging is preferred because post-processing from isotropic voxels creates sharp images while anisotropic voxels may create images that are not as distinct. Spiral CT creates two-dimensional images oriented in an axial plane. The resolution is high and image reconstruction is almost isotropic, which is optimized by selecting a reconstruction increment of 50% of the slice thickness, which increases the spatial resolution in the z-axis. The parameters for image reconstruction in CT coronary angiography typically are slice thickness of 1 mm (ideally less), reconstruction increment 0.5 mm (or less) and FOV 150 mm. Post-processing imaging is performed from a three-dimensional data set that is reconstructed from the obtained axial images, which should always be considered as the source information of CT imaging (Figure 2.2). The three-dimensional data set can be reformatted according to the needs of the investigator using several types of post-processing algorithms (Table 2.1).

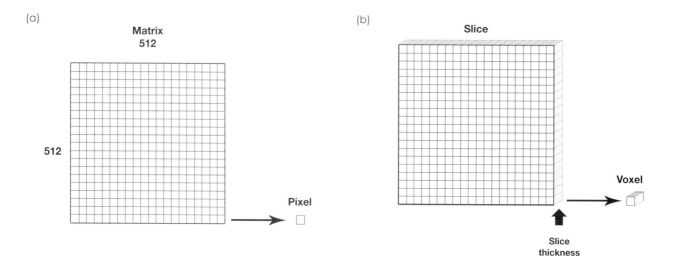

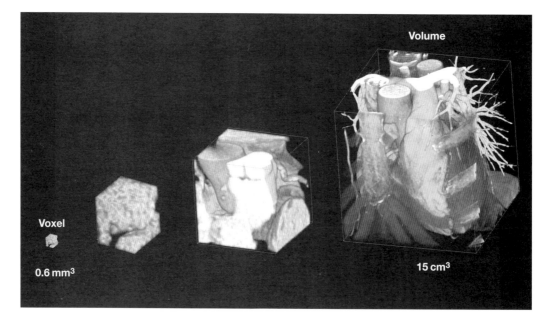

Figure 2.1 The matrix of the image represents the number of pixels that are by convention used for the reconstruction (a). In all current CT images the matrix is 512×512 pixels (262 144 pixels). The matrix is constant and is not affected by the size of the field of view. The field of view can be varied and in cardiac CT imaging it usually ranges around 150 mm. The size of the field of view affects the size of the pixel. For instance, for a field of view of 150 mm, the pixel in the matrix will be 0.3 mm². When a slice is reconstructed, a third dimension is added to the matrix. This dimension corresponds to the slice thickness and depends mainly on the collimation (b). Ideally, the slice thickness should be in the range of the size of the pixel in the matrix (i.e. 0.3 mm² for a field of view of 150 mm). When this requirement is met, the voxel is called isotropic. (c) Voxel and volume

POST-PROCESSING TECHNIQUES

Axial image scrolling

The axial images are considered to be the source images providing the basic information in CT. Scrolling through these images in the cranio–caudal direction allows interpretation of the cardiac structures including the coronary arteries (Figure 2.3). However, because of the complex course of the coronary arteries interpretation of the axial images may be difficult and better insight may be obtained from multiplanar reconstructions.

Multiplanar reconstruction

Multiplanar reconstructions (MPRs) can be generated from the volume data set which is reconstructed from a

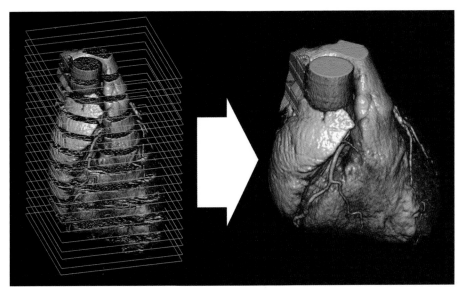

Figure 2.2 The source information of CT is the axial images. The axial images are reconstructed with a defined x-y-z resolution. This stack of images is reconstructed to form a volume. Post-processing is performed on this volume data set

Table 2.1 Post-processing techniques

Axial image scrolling

Multiplanar reconstructions (MPR)

Curved multiplanar reconstructions (cMPR)

Maximum intensity projections (MIP)

Shaded surface display (SSD)

Three-dimensional volume rendering (VR)

Virtual endoscopy (VE)

Vessel analysis (VA) and vessel tracking (VT)

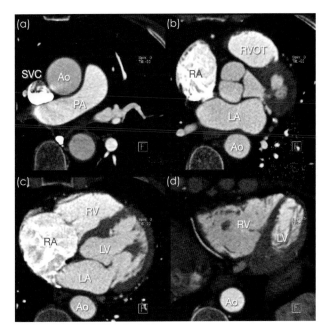

Figure 2.3 Axial images. The axial images are the basic information of the CT scanner. Scrolling through them in the cranial to caudal direction will show the structures of interest in the axial plane. Usually a cardiac CT scan starts at the level of the main stem of the pulmonary artery (PA) where the ascending aorta (Ao) and superior vena cava (SVC) run orthogonal to the scan plane (a). At the level of the aortic valve both atria are visualized as well as the outflow tract of the right ventricle (RVOT) (b). More inferior, the four cardiac chambers are displayed (c). Finally, the inferior side of the heart is shown with the distal right coronary artery and the inferior walls of the right and left ventricle (LV) (d). The aorta descendens is visualized in (b), (c) and (d). RA, right atrium, LA, left atrium; RV, right ventricle

stack of axial images (Figure 2.4)[3]. In principle, any plane can be generated from the volume data set, but by convention the most often used relevant planes in routine radiology are the axial, sagittal and coronal planes (Figure 2.4), while oblique planes may also be useful. Planes that are oriented parallel or orthogonal to the interventricular or atrioventricular grooves are very useful in coronary MPRs.

The slice thickness can be modified to create a 'thick slab', which may be useful to visualize (a part of) a tortuous coronary artery. The advantages of MPR are: (1) that it is a relatively simple algorithm which can be rendered quickly and accurately on any image-processing workstations without the need of segmentation of overlapping structures; (2) distance measurements in MPR

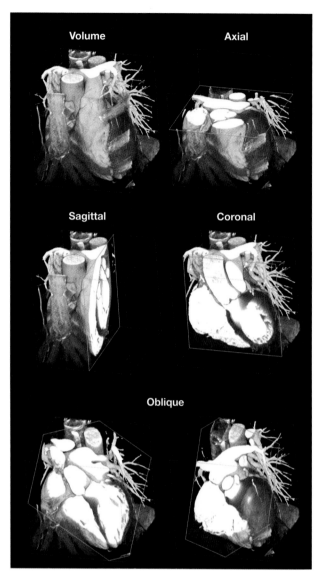

Figure 2.4 Multiplanar reconstructions are generated from the interpolation of the stack of axial images into a volume of data (Volume). The conventional planes that are used for visualization are the axial plane (Axial), the sagittal plane (Sagittal) and the coronal plane (Coronal). These planes should be imagined as slices that cut the volume with a defined spatial orientation. The cut planes can be arbitrarily tilted in any orientation to create orthogonal or parallel planes through the structures of interest (Oblique)

are accurate and not subject to foreshortening; (3) different structures in MPR are accurate and do not overlap; and (4) 100% of the available data is represented in the images (no loss of voxel value information due to thresholding). A disadvantage of MPR is that the image quality is highly dependent on the resolution and isotropy of the data volume set.

Curved multiplanar reconstruction imaging

Curved MPR (cMPR) is defined as a plane that is reformatted along a curved plane. Curved MPRs are useful for the visualization of coronary arteries where a curved MPR is reconstructed along the curved course of the coronary artery of interest (Figure 2.5). This enables the entire coronary artery to be followed and displayed in one reconstruction. The curved MPR planes tend to distort the actual configuration of the anatomical structures that are represented in the volume. It is recommended that at least two images in orthogonal planes are reconstructed to prevent under- or overestimation of the severity of coronary lesions.

Maximum intensity projection

Maximum intensity projection (MIP) is a projectional technique. Imaging rays are cast through the three-dimensional data volume from the viewpoint of the user, and only the highest-intensity voxels encountered by each ray are used to reconstruct the two-dimensional projection image (Figure 2.6)[3,4]. It resembles the principle of conventional angiography because the result is a projection of the highest attenuation values on the image. MIP vascular imaging allows differentiation between enhanced vascular structures and non-vascular structures and, because most of the volume data are discarded, it requires a relatively short reconstruction time. A potential problem with MIP is that superimposed higher-density structures obscure the lower-density structures of interest, which is the case when calcium is present along the imaginary ray from the observer point of view. This problem can be avoided by using a limited stack of images (e.g. a 'slab') with a thickness adjusted to the size and course of the coronary arteries (Figure 2.6). Another problem is that MIP images lack 'depth' information, which fortunately does not play a significant role in coronary artery imaging.

Shaded surface display

Shaded surface display (SSD) is a three-dimensional technique that recreates a surface of an object using contour information based on a selected threshold of the voxel within the volume data set (Figure 2.7). All the voxels above or below the preselected threshold form a

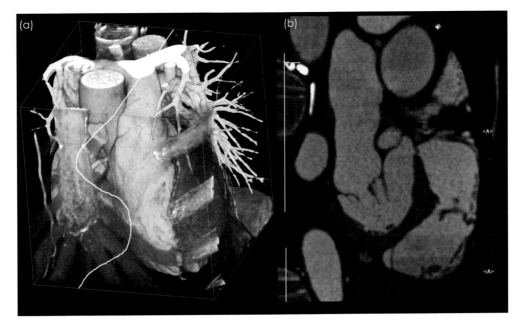

Figure 2.5 Curved multiplanar reconstructions are generated by means of flat planes that cut the volume with a defined spatial orientation. When the cut plane is not flat, but instead is curved, the result is a curved multiplanar reconstruction (a). The main difference compared with conventional multiplanar reconstructions is that the resulting image is a flattened representation of the curved plane (b). In this image the geometric relationships are less consistent

solid surface. To improve the three-dimensional impression, a simulated light source is added to provide shading effects.

SSD provides no density information, implying that calcifications or contrast-enhanced coronary lumen are presented in the same way[4,5]. Typically SSD uses only 10% of the available volume data and is now replaced by three-dimensional volume rendering which uses 100% of the available volume data.

Three-dimensional volume rendering

Three-dimensional volume rendering uses all the voxels of the volume data to create a three-dimensional image based on the density of each voxel[1,3,6]. Volume rendering requires pre-processing tissue types contained in each voxel. The voxels are classified according to the density value of major tissues: air, fat, soft tissue and bone. Air has a density of $-1000\,HU$, fat approximately $-100\,HU$, soft tissue $+50\,HU$ and bone $+1000\,HU$ (Figure 2.8). Volume rendering assigns a certain opacity to each voxel density value to make some structures opaque and others transparent. Lowering the opacity of the voxel values which are not of interest causes the corresponding voxels to become transparent, while increasing the opacity causes these structures to become more opaque. The settings of the opacity function can be fully adapted to meet the requirements of the observer (Figure 2.9). In addition a color can be assigned to the classified voxels representing different tissues (Figure 2.10). The default setting for bone is yellowish white and for soft tissue is reddish brown. The default opacity setting is high for bone, medium to low for soft tissue, and fat and air are fully transparent. When processing the opacity value is set high for the tissues of interest and low for other tissues. It is of note that different settings may affect the appearance of a structure, and may have an effect on the size of the (in particular smaller) coronary vessels (Figure 2.11).

Virtual endoscopy

The concept of virtual endoscopy was first introduced in the context of the visualization of the inner surface of hollow organs. The main applications are in the colon (Figure 2.12), airways (Figure 2.13), stomach and bladder. In virtual endoscopy the air within the colon is made transparent to create a virtual space within the

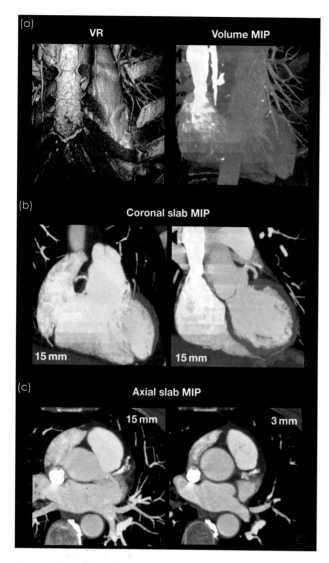

Figure 2.6 Maximum intensity projections (MIPs) are projectional images that visualize only the voxel with the highest attenuation along the observation line. The perception of depth is completely lost when MIPs are applied to a volume of data, especially if compared to volume rendering (VR) (a). MIP reconstructions are more effective and informative when applied to thick slabs of images (b) and (c)

colon. The surrounding tissues have a different attenuation (e.g. higher or lower) and are made opaque. Thus, the surface of the walls of the colon is created from the point of view of the observer positioned inside the colon.

Virtual bronchoscopy uses the same technique (Figure 2.13). This concept applied to vascular imaging produces a virtual angioscopic visualization (Figure 2.14) of the arteries. The very dense contrast material inside the vessel is made transparent and the walls of the

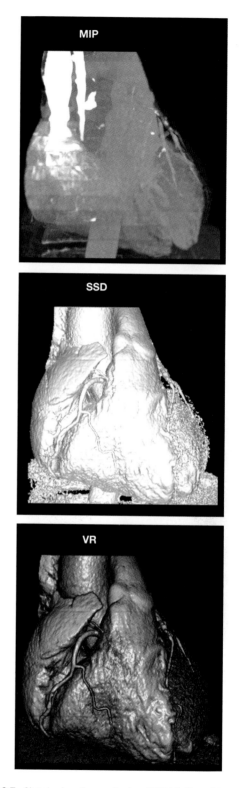

Figure 2.7 Shaded surface display (SSD) is the oldest of the three-dimensional techniques. The technique shows a surface of an object based on the selection of a threshold. It gives more depth information when compared to volumetric maximum intensity projections (MIP), but is very limited when compared to volume rendering (VR)

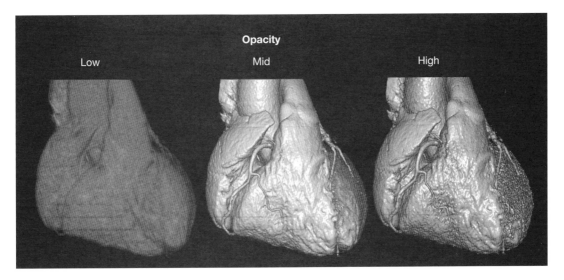

Figure 2.8 Volume rendering: opacity. The opacity (or transparency) is assigned to a voxel in order to allow the observer to see through it or to make it completely opaque. In the figure a volume of data is displayed with increasing opacity from left to right

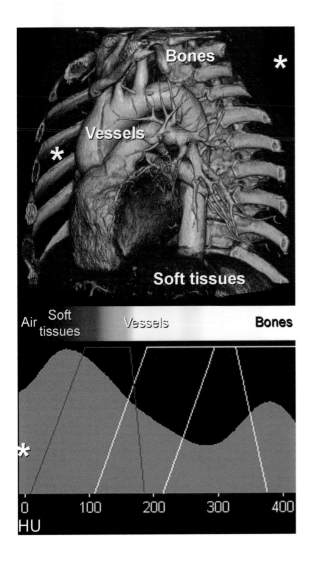

Figure 2.9 Volume rendering is a three-dimensional technique that displays the voxels of the volume based on the density. In addition, a value of opacity can be assigned to each voxel in order to let the observer look through defined ranges of attenuation. The opacity settings can be arbitrarily selected according to the requirements of the observer. In this example, the range of attenuation below 0 HU (fat, lung parenchyma and air) are transparent (asterisk). The soft tissue with a range of attenuation between 0 and 180 HU (subcutaneous tissue, liver parenchyma and myocardium) are assigned the color red. The tissues with a range of attenuation between 110 and 370 HU (vessels) are assigned a yellow color. The tissues with attenuation above 220 HU (bones) are assigned the color white. The color stripe in the middle of the image shows the progressive change of color along the scale of attenuation

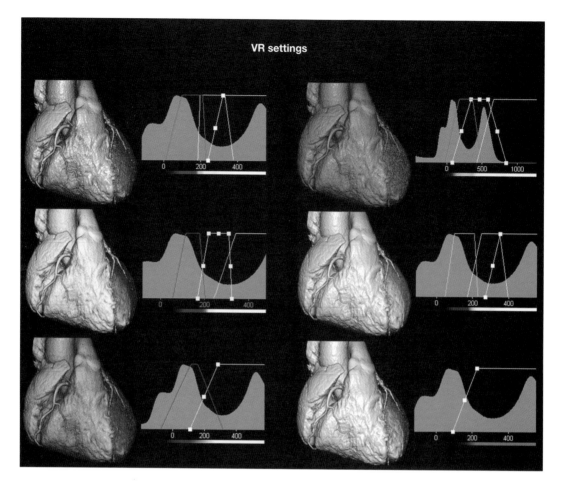

Figure 2.10 Volume rendering (VR): color attribution. In VR the parameters attributed to an image are arbitrary. Therefore, the appearance will change when the operator changes the colors of the algorithm

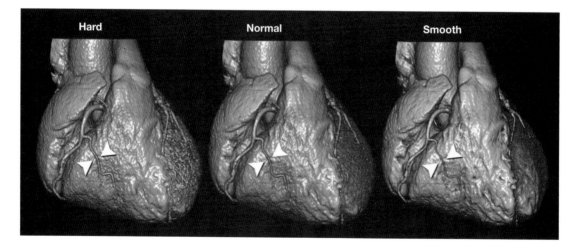

Figure 2.11 Volume rendering (VR) and vessel diameter. VR is based on arbitrary settings and modification of these settings may affect the size of the vessels. This is particularly evident for small vessels such as coronary arteries. The image shows how the diameter of a marginal branch of the right coronary artery (arrowheads) can be modified by the application of progressively smoother VR settings

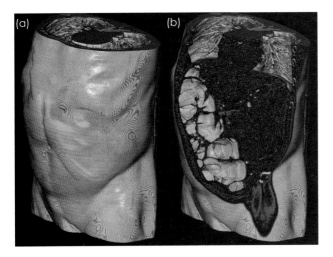

Figure 2.12 Virtual colonoscopy is based on the visualization of the colon as a hollow organ after the inflation of air. The volume of data is made opaque (a) and the air is made transparent (b) and the walls of the colon are also made opaque. A surface is generated and the abnormalities of the surface, such as polyps, can be easily detected

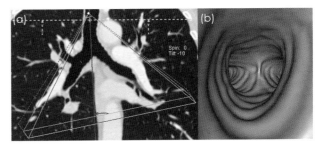

Figure 2.13 Virtual bronchoscopy is based on the same principles as virtual colonoscopy. The air inside the airways is made transparent while the walls of the trachea are opaque. A point of view inside the trachea is chosen (a) and the surface of the airways can be displayed as with fiberoptic bronchoscopy (b). The main applications of this technique are to detect upper airway abnormalities, e.g. carcinoma

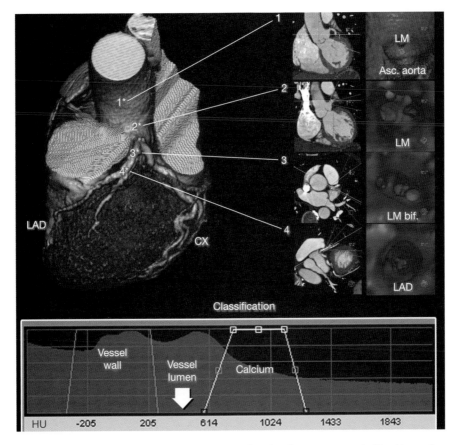

Figure 2.14 Virtual angioscopy is based on the same principle as virtual colonoscopy and virtual bronchoscopy. The contrast material inside the vessel lumen is made transparent and the vessel wall is made orange and the calcium white (see the lower part of the figure). Virtual angioscopy is applied from the ascending (Asc.) aorta and the coronary arteries. The point of view of the observer is within the vessel and is progressing from the ascending aorta (1), to the ostium of the left main coronary artery (LM) (2), the bifurcation of left main (LM bif.) (3), to the left anterior descending (LAD) (4). LCX, left circumflex

vessels are made opaque. This technique produces spectacular images but, so far, its clinical use is limited.

Vessel analysis and vessel tracking

Segmentation involves the simplification of an image by dividing it into its basic component elements or objects. Segmentation can be done in several ways such as vessel tracking, contouring, region growing, etc. Segmentation of the vessels by vessel tracking is a fast semi-automated or even fully automated software algorithm which significantly reduces the often time-consuming task of post-processing[7].

Segmentation of vessels is based on density, spatial geometry and homogeneity of the vessel structure within the volume data set[6,8,9]. Vessel segmentation is a necessary step preceding quantitative vessel-lumen analysis using contour-detection algorithms. With vessel tracking software, a central lumen line can be generated simply by positioning a beginning and endpoint in the vessel region of interest. The lumen contours of the vessel are determined by contour-detection algorithms taking the central lumen line as the starting point. Thus, a cross-sectional contour of the vessel is generated, which allows quantification of the vessel lumen (Figure 2.15). Various software packages are available, but it is extremely difficult to produce an accurate and reliable algorithm for the coronary arteries which are small, have a tortuous course and the image quality obtained by CT is not always optimal for automated construction of a central lumen line and lumen contour detection.

Post-processing techniques in clinical practice

Which, when and how to use the various available post-processing techniques remains a matter of personal experience and may differ amongst various operators. In

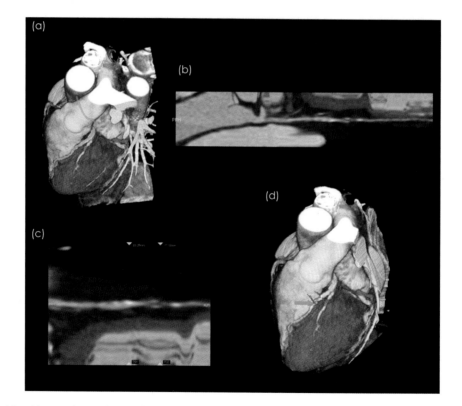

Figure 2.15 Vessel tracking and vessel analysis. The first step is to track the path of the vessel. The operator selects two points: one at the beginning and one at the end of the vessel, which allows the software to identify the path of the vessel (a). The software then creates a stretched curved multiplanar reconstruction along the central lumen line (b). This longitudinal view can be rotated around its axis to evaluate the position of the branches and the location and longitudinal extent of plaques (c). In the longitudinal view automated lumen measurements can be performed and their position is easily indicated on the three-dimensional volume rendering (d)

Table 2.2 we present the advantages and disadvantages of the available techniques. Table 2.3 is a summary of our experience using the various post-processing techniques in clinical practice. The techniques were scored according to a range of variables:

(1) Availability. The availability of post-processing techniques is inversely proportional to their computational complexity. All DICOM (Digital Imaging and Communication in Medicine) viewing software allows axial images to be scrolled, while for increasingly complex tasks, such as MPR, MIP and volume rendering, more sophisticated software and computer power are required.

(2) Reliability. The reliability of the technique represents how the information displayed reflects the original data after the algorithm is applied.

(3) Experience. The experience required to use these techniques is dependent on the type of training. Radiologists are used to interaction with cross-sectional images and will feel comfortable using the technique, while a cardiologist, not by training familiar with the technique, might require additional education. Even though the techniques that show three-dimensional anatomical configuration, such as volume rendering, provide information that is easier to understand, some experience is required to handle the data properly.

(4) Time. The time needed to obtain relevant images is also dependent on the training of the operator and on the complexity of the technique and, even more, on whether the output is qualitative (e.g. images) or quantitative (e.g. stenosis assessment).

(5) Diagnosis. The impact of each post-processing technique is different. For the assessment of stenoses and plaques the techniques that show the original data in planes favorable to coronary anatomy (e.g. axial scrolling, MPR, cMPR and MIP) are preferred. With these images the real densitometric information can be evaluated.

Table 2.2 Comparison of post-processing techniques

Technique	Advantages	Disadvantages
Axial scrolling	true data artefacts easily recognized anatomical overview	no three-dimensional perception
MPR	true data artifacts easily recognized anatomical overview vessel area measurement	poor three-dimensional perception
cMPR	complete overview of the vessel of interest	highly operator dependent no anatomical overview time-consuming requires two or more orthogonal projections
MIP	partial overview of the vessel of interest	over-projection of calcium and stents no visualization of vessel wall requires at least two orthogonal projections
SSD	overview and orientation	user dependent no visualization of vessel wall poor evaluation of stents and calcium
VR	three-dimensional perception complete anatomical overview relation to myocardium	user-dependent no visualization of vessel wall poor evaluation of stents and calcium time-consuming
VE	none	user dependent no visualization of vessel wall no anatomical overview

MPR, multiplanar reconstructions; cMPR, curved multiplanar reconstructions; MIP, maximum intensity projections; SSD, shaded surface display; VR, volume rendering; VE, virtual endoscopy; VA, vessel analysis; VT, vessel tracking

Table 2.3 Post-processing techniques: impact and role in cardiac CT

Technique	Availability	Reliability	Experience	Time	Diagnosis Stenosis plaques	CABG	Others*	Presentation	Communication
Axial scrolling	high	high	low	low	low	low	high	low	low
MPR	high	high	low	low	high	high	high	low	low
cMPR	mid	high	mid	low	high	high	mid	mid	high
MIP	mid	mid	mid	low	mid	high	high	mid	high
SSD	mid	low	mid	mid	low	low	low	low	low
VR	mid	low	high	mid	low	high	mid	high	high
VE	low	low	high	high	low	low	low	mid	low
VA and VT	low	?	high	high	high?	high?	?	high	?

*Others relates to cardiac CT performed for non-coronary purposes. The question marks in the VA and VT are due to the still limited experience and validation of automatic or semi-automatic tools for vessel tracking and evaluation.

CABG, coronary artery bypass graft; MPR, multiplanar reconstructions; cMPR, curved multiplanar reconstructions; MIP, maximum intensity projections; SSD, shaded surface display; VR, volume rendering; VE, virtual endoscopy; VA, vessel analysis; VT, vessel tracking

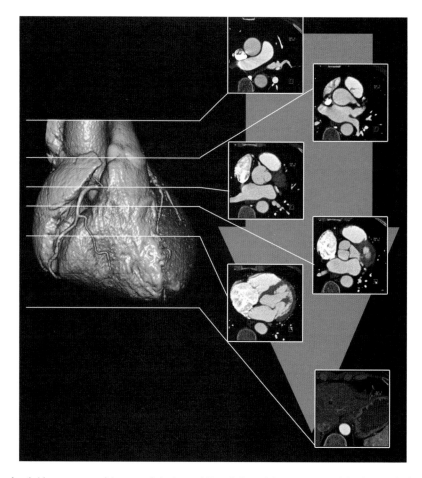

Figure 2.16 Scrolling of axial images provides a quick view of the data set to assess crudely the main features of the coronary anatomy. When scrolling the images the observer should create in his mind a quick roadmap of the main features of the patient's vessels

Volume rendering is used in coronary artery bypass graft evaluation to understand better the anatomical configuration of the grafts. In other non-coronary applications the diagnostic information should be evaluated on axial and multi-planar images.

(6) Presentation and communication. For presentation and communication purposes the axial and multiplanar images are less informative because they presuppose interaction with the volume which is difficult to display in a still frame.

Post-processing protocol

At the beginning of each evaluation an overview of the data set should be performed to detect gross abnormalities, artifacts and the presence of extracoronary and myocardial abnormalities. To analyze coronary arteries a systematic approach should be followed. It is recommended that the coronary segments are evaluated in a sequential order from segment 1 to segment 15 following the standard report of the American Heart Association.

Protocol

Axial images should always be reviewed first (Figure 2.16). Scrolling axial images up and down will allow all the non-coronary information to be reviewed that might be present within the data set. At the same time the location of cardiac structures (e.g. great vessels of the thorax, cardiac valves, atria, ventricles), including coronary arteries, can be screened for gross morphological abnormalities. After scrolling of axial images the observer should shift to MPR (Figure 2.17). With this technique dedicated planes can be generated to represent better coronary segments or entire coronary vessels.

There are two main planes (Figure 2.18) that are useful for the evaluation of coronary arteries:

(1) The plane for the right coronary artery and the left circumflex artery is parallel to the atrio-

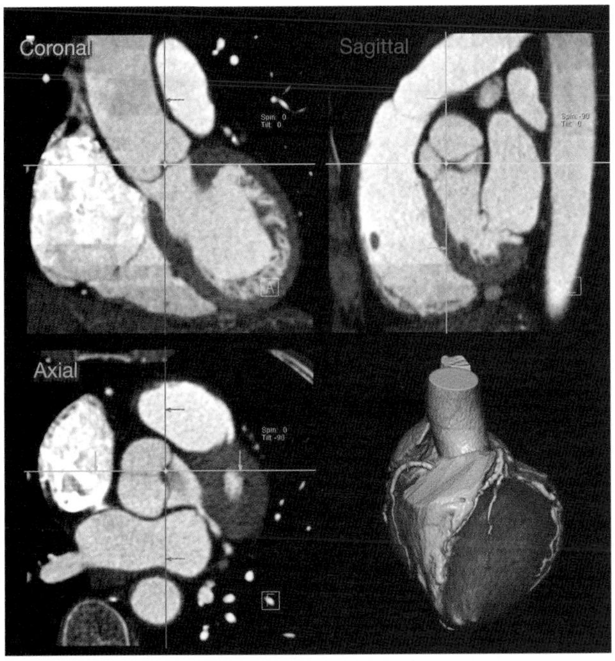

Figure 2.17 Scrolling multiplanar reconstructions. After scrolling the axial images the observer should use multiplanar reconstructions to orientate better the planes of visualization to the geometrical orientation of the coronary structures. The starting planes, as previously described, are the axial, coronal and sagittal planes (see Figure 2.4)

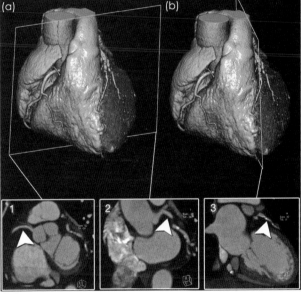

Figure 2.18 Multiplanar reconstruction planes for the coronary arteries. The planes that can help to visualize better the coronary arteries are a plane parallel to the atrioventricular groove (a) and a plane parallel to the interventricular groove (b). The first plane shows the right coronary artery (1) and the left circumflex (2). The second plane shows the left anterior descending artery (3). The tortuous anatomy of the left coronary artery most of the time does not allow the entire vessel to be represented in a single image

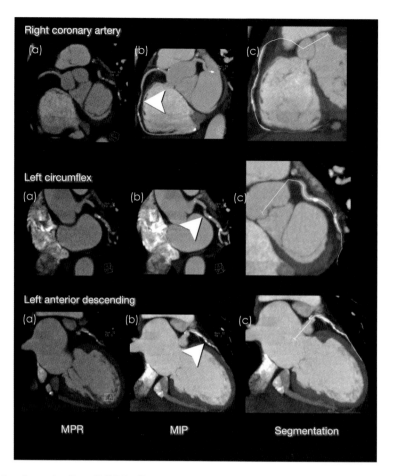

Figure 2.19 Maximum intensity projections (MIP) for the coronary arteries. Multiplanar reconstructions (MPR) can be used to set the cut planes in an orientation that matches one of the main coronary arteries. Nevertheless, the tortuous anatomy of coronary vessels does not allow the complete visualization of the vessel in many cases (a). The use of maximum intensity projections can increase the overview for each vessel (b). Using maximum intensity projections it is also easier to track the path of the vessel when performing curved multiplanar reconstructions (c)

ventricular groove and can be defined as a para-coronal plane. Scrolling the plane on this axis the observer can follow the path of the right coronary artery and the left circumflex. Sometimes the ideal plane for the right coronary artery is slightly different to that for the left circumflex artery.

(2) The plane for the left anterior descending artery is parallel to the interventricular septum and can be defined as a parasagittal plane. The vessel can be followed easily by scrolling these planes back and forth. When calcifications are not too prominent the application of a slab MIP, 3–5 mm thick, allows the entire vessel or most of it to be projected in the same image (Figure 2.19). Following the vessel throughout the optimal plane and manually or automatically tracing the central-

lumen line will result in a single image representing the entire vessel (Figure 2.20). In order to obtain the orthogonal projection of this image, the tracing of the central-lumen line should be performed on a plane orthogonal to the one previously described, or, when automatic, the vessel should be rotated 360° around its axis. When lesions or suspected lesions are detected, the segment of interest should be magnified and a plane orthogonal to the path of the vessel should be used for the evaluation (Figure 2.21). Scrolling back and forth along the axis of the lumen the observer will be able to evaluate the patency of the vessel, looking first at the proximal non-diseased region and then focusing the image on the diseased region. At the end of the evaluation

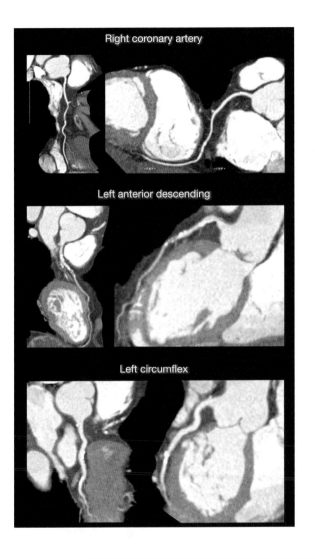

Figure 2.20 Curved multiplanar reconstructions for the coronary arteries. Coronary arteries have a tortuous anatomy; therefore, it can be difficult to show the entire vessel in one image. An easy way to do this is by means of curved multiplanar reconstructions. The vessel is segmented using multiplanar planes with or without maximum intensity projections (see Figure 2.19). Then the resulting image is projected into one plane. From two orthogonal planes the observer can have a quick overview of the vessel anatomy and abnormalities

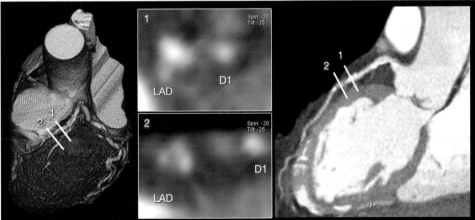

Figure 2.21 Orthogonal views for the coronary arteries. When abnormalities are detected in the lumen or in the wall of coronary arteries, the observer can always create a plane orthogonal to the direction of the vessel. This view, which is commonly used in intravascular ultrasound, allows the configuration of the disease along the vessel to be seen. In the figure, two orthogonal views (1 and 2) are performed at the level of segment 7 (mid left anterior descending) immediately after the bifurcation of the first diagonal. The first view (1) is performed at the level of normal lumen, while the second view (2) is performed at the level of a significant (> 50%) lumen reduction in the left anterior descending (LAD). D1, first diagonal

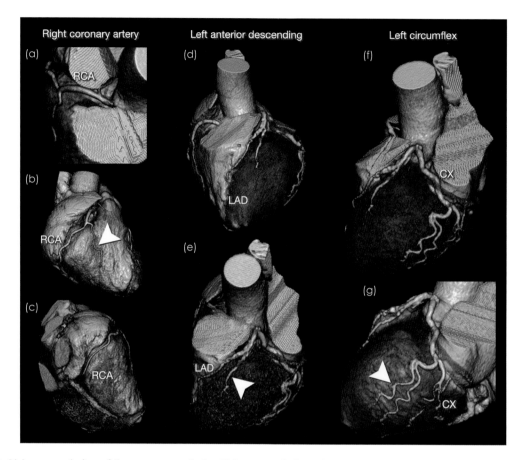

Figure 2.22 Volume rendering of the coronary arteries. Volume rendering allows an easy overview of coronary artery anatomy. It does not allow quantitative or semi-quantitative evaluations regarding the patency of the lumen of the arteries to be performed. Nevertheless, it assists significantly in understanding the topography of coronary vessels and the position of the lesions in the coronary tree. Dedicated projections for each of the three main vessels are performed. The proximal segment of the right coronary artery (RCA) is visualized in a cranial view (a). The mid-segment of the RCA (b) is visualized in a view from the right side in which a marginal branch is clearly shown (arrowhead). The distal segment of the RCA is visualized in a right caudal view (c). The left anterior descending (LAD) is visualized in a left anterior view (d) and a cranial left view (e) where the first diagonal branch is visualized (arrowhead). The left circumflex artery (CX) is visualized in a left cranial view (f) and a left view (g) where several marginal branches are clearly displayed (arrowhead)

a volume rendering can be performed to give an anatomical picture of the coronary arteries and to create images useful for the report (Figure 2.22).

REPORTING

A report for coronary CT angiography (CTA) should be similar to that of a conventional coronary angiography report (Figure 2.23). A report should be based on a visual approach with clear reference to the segment with disease. Particular attention should be given to calcification and motion artifacts that may impair the visualization of the vessels.

CORONARY ARTERY BYPASS GRAFT EVALUATION

Volume rendering should be used prior to other post-processing techniques to give an overview of the entire anatomy, which is often helpful to understand the anatomy of the grafts (Figure 2.24).

NON-CORONARY STUDIES

Axial and MPR images are recommended to detect non-coronary abnormalities.

(a)

Cardiac MSCT

Name:	Contrast typ.:	mgl/ml	mAs:
Birth:	Contrast vol.:	ml	kV
ID:	Contrast rate:	ml/s	Coll:
Date:	Metroprolol:	mg	Slices:
	HR:	bpm	Rot. Time:

Referring physician:	....
History:	....
	....
Clinical question:	....

Coronary angiography

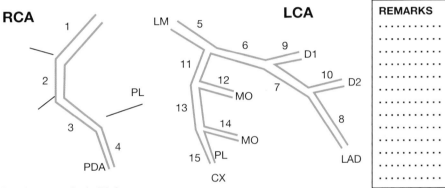

Dominant   Left–Right

Seg.	Vessel	Patent	Stenosis	Conf$^\alpha$	Small	Qual$^\beta$	Stent	Calcium
01	RCA	Y – N	0 /<50 / ±50 />50 / NA	1-2-3	...	1-2-3	...	0 / + / ++
02	RCA	Y – N	0 /<50 / ±50 />50 / NA	1-2-3	...	1-2-3	...	0 / + / ++
03	RCA	Y – N	0 /<50 / ±50 />50 / NA	1-2-3	...	1-2-3	...	0 / + / ++
04	PDA	Y – N	0 /<50 / ±50 />50 / NA	1-2-3	...	1-2-3	...	0 / + / ++
05	LM	Y – N	0 /<50 / ±50 />50 / NA	1-2-3	...	1-2-3	...	0 / + / ++
06	LAD	Y – N	0 /<50 / ±50 />50 / NA	1-2-3	...	1-2-3	...	0 / + / ++
07	LAD	Y – N	0 /<50 / ±50 />50 / NA	1-2-3	...	1-2-3	...	0 / + / ++
08	LAD	Y – N	0 /<50 / ±50 />50 / NA	1-2-3	...	1-2-3	...	0 / + / ++
09	D1	Y – N	0 /<50 / ±50 />50 / NA	1-2-3	...	1-2-3	...	0 / + / ++
10	D2	Y – N	0 /<50 / ±50 />50 / NA	1-2-3	...	1-2-3	...	0 / + / ++
11	CX	Y – N	0 /<50 / ±50 />50 / NA	1-2-3	...	1-2-3	...	0 / + / ++
12	MO	Y – N	0 /<50 / ±50 />50 / NA	1-2-3	...	1-2-3	...	0 / + / ++
13	CX	Y – N	0 /<50 / ±50 />50 / NA	1-2-3	...	1-2-3	...	0 / + / ++
14	MO	Y – N	0 /<50 / ±50 />50 / NA	1-2-3	...	1-2-3	...	0 / + / ++
15	PL	Y – N	0 /<50 / ±50 />50 / NA	1-2-3	...	1-2-3	...	0 / + / ++

α = non-reliable, 2 = moderately reliable, 3 = reliable
β 1 = poor, 2 = adequate, 3 = good

Figure 2.23 Example of a reporting form for cardiac CT. The general CT report should assess coronary angiography, coronary calcium score and overview of the heart. (a) Coronary angiography: coronary arteries are evaluated following the standard segmental classification of the American Heart Association. Each segment should be scored as normal, < 50% obstruction, > 50% obstruction or total occlusion. Sometimes the segment is not assessable (NA) because of several reasons: too small, too calcified or motion artifact. In addition, a confidence level is assigned to the assessment as well as the quality of the image. The presence of stents should be noted and a visual score for calcium (absent = 0; nodules = +; bulk = ++) should be performed. (b) Coronary calcium: the calcium score is given as the Agatston, volume and mass score. The calcium score (in quartiles) is presented for age and gender, and general guidelines are given for interpretation of the calcium score. (c) Left ventricle: evaluation of left ventricular function and motion abnormalities. The presence of additional cardiac and non-cardiac abnormalities should be noted

(b)

Coronary calcium score

Calcium score

	RCA	LM	LAD	CX	Total
Agatston	....	....	....	....	....
Volume (mm^3)	....	....	....	....	....
Mass (mg)	....	....	....	....	....

CALCIUM SCORE										
Gender	Perc.	Age (years)								
		<40	40–44	45–49	50–54	55–59	60–64	65–69	70–74	>74
Men	25th	0	0	0	1	4	13	32	64	166
	50th	1	1	3	15	48	113	180	310	473
	75th	3	9	36	103	215	410	566	892	1071
	90th	14	59	154	332	554	994	1299	1774	1982
	n.	3504	4238	4940	4825	3472	2288	1209	540	235
Women	25th	0	0	0	0	0	0	1	3	9
	50th	0	0	0	0	1	3	24	52	75
	75th	1	1	2	5	23	57	145	210	241
	90th	3	4	22	55	121	193	410	631	709
	n.	641	1024	1634	2184	1835	1334	731	438	174

Reproduced from Hoff JA et al. JACC 2003;41:1008–12.

General Guidelines for Interpretation of Calcium Score			
Calcium Score*	Atherosclerotic plaque burden	Probability of significant CAD	Implications for CV risk
0	No detectable plaque	Very low (<5%)	Very low
1–10	Minimal detectable plaque burden	Very unlikely (<10%)	Low
11–100	Mild atherosclerotic plaque burden	Mild or minimal	Moderate
101–400	Moderate atherosclerotic plaque burden	High likelihood of non-obstructive CAD Possibility of obstructive disease	Moderately high
>400	Extensive atherosclerotic plaque burden	High likelihood of one or more 'significant' obstructive lesions (>90%)	High

Modified from Rumberger JA et al. Mayo Clinic Proc 1999;74:243–252.
*Values in the Table should be age/gender adjusted.

REMARKS

. . . .
. . . .
. . . .
. . . .
. . . .

Figure 2.23 *continued* (see legend on page 43)

(c)

Left ventricle

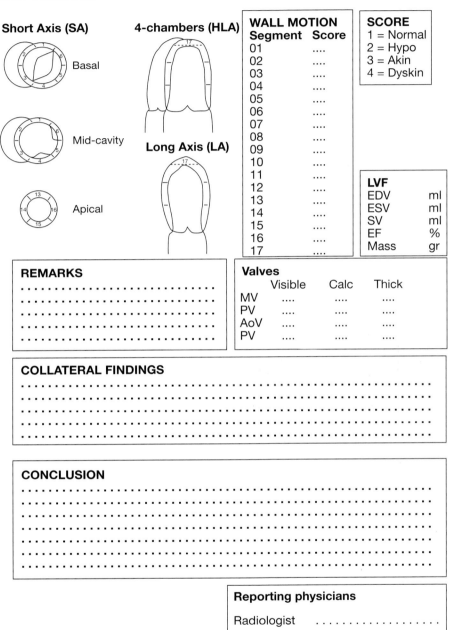

REMARKS

....
....
....
....
....

Valves

	Visible	Calc	Thick
MV	....	....	....
PV	....	....	....
AoV	....	....	....
PV	....	....	....

COLLATERAL FINDINGS

....
....
....
....
....
....

CONCLUSION

....
....
....
....
....
....
....

Reporting physicians

Radiologist ....

Cardiologist ....

Figure 2.23 *continued* (see legend on page 43)

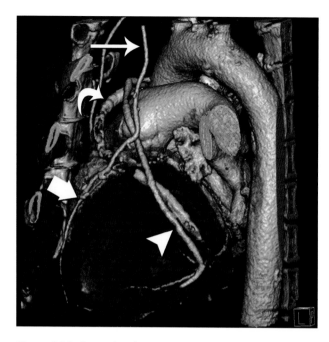

Figure 2.24 Example of a coronary artery bypass graft. The anatomical configuration of the coronary artery bypass graft can be better evaluated with three-dimensional volume rendering. In the case of coronary artery bypass grafts, the native coronary arteries (left anterior descending, thick arrow) are crossed by other vessels, such as the left internal mammary artery (thin arrow) and the saphenous vein grafts, one of which is patent (arrowhead), the other is occluded (curved arrow)

REFERENCES

1. Calhoun PS, Kuszyk BS, Heath DG, et al. Three-dimensional volume rendering of spiral CT data: theory and method. Radiographics 1999; 19: 745–64

2. Fishman EK, Magid D, Ney DR, et al. Three-dimensional imaging. Radiology 1991; 181: 321–37

3. Lichtenbelt B, Crane R, Naqvi S. Introduction to volume rendering. Hewlett-Packard Professional Books. Upper Saddle River, NJ: Prentice Hall PTR, 1998

4. Semba CP, Rubin GD, Dake MD. Three-dimensional spiral CT angiography of the abdomen. Semin Ultrasound CT MR 1994; 15: 133–8

5. Sato Y, Shiraga N, Nakajima S, et al. Local maximum intensity projection (LMIP): a new rendering method for vascular visualization. J Comput Assist Tomogr 1998; 22: 912–17

6. Udupa JK. Three-dimensional visualization and analysis methodologies: a current perspective. Radiographics 1999; 19: 783–806

7. Hohne KH, Hanson WA. Interactive 3D segmentation of MRI and CT volumes using morphological operations. J Comput Assist Tomogr 1992; 16: 285–94

8. Masutani Y, MacMahon H, Doi K. Automated segmentation and visualization of the pulmonary vascular tree in spiral CT angiography: an anatomy-oriented approach based on three-dimensional image analysis. J Comput Assist Tomogr 2001; 25: 587–97

9. Clarke LP, Velthuizen RP, Camacho MA, et al. MRI segmentation: methods and applications. Magn Reson Imaging 1995; 13: 343–68

CHAPTER 3

Coronary imaging: normal coronary anatomy

Volume-rendered CT cardiac images resemble the gross anatomy of the heart and provide a precise anatomical presentation of the presence and course of the right and left coronary arteries in relation to the surrounding cardiac structures. The coronary arteries are presented in a three-dimensional fashion, and as cross-sectional images. Superimposed structures, such as the atria and appendages, the pulmonary trunk and cardiac veins can obscure the view and are preferably removed.

CORONARY ANATOMY

The left main coronary artery arises from the left posterior aortic sinus. It varies in length, but is usually 1–2 cm (Figure 3.1). In a small proportion of cases the left main coronary artery is very short and bifurcates almost immediately. In 0.41% of cases the left main coronary artery does not develop, and the left anterior descending and circumflex arteries each arise individually from in the left coronary sinus. The main left coronary artery bifurcates, beneath the left atrial appendage, into the left anterior descending (LAD) and the circumflex arteries (Figure 3.2). The LAD artery passes to the left of the pulmonary trunk and turns forwards to run downwards in the anterior interventricular groove (Figure 3.2). The LAD artery provides two main groups of branches: first, the septal branches, which supply the anterior two-thirds of the septum and, second, the diagonal branches which lie on the lateral aspect of the left ventricle. The circumflex artery turns backwards shortly beyond its origin to run downwards in the left atrioventricular groove. It, too, gives rise to a variable number of marginal branches, which run on and supply the lateral aspect of the left ventricle. In the atrioventricular groove the circumflex artery is often covered by the auri-

cle of the left atrium, which obstructs visualization and therefore has to be removed from the data set. In one-third of subjects the left main coronary artery trifurcates into the LAD, left circumflex and an intermediate artery, which follows a course between the circumflex and LAD arteries over the anterolateral wall of the left ventricle.

The right coronary artery (RCA) arises from the anterior aortic sinus, passes forwards and then downwards, in the right atrioventricular groove, and continues around the margin of the heart towards the crux, a

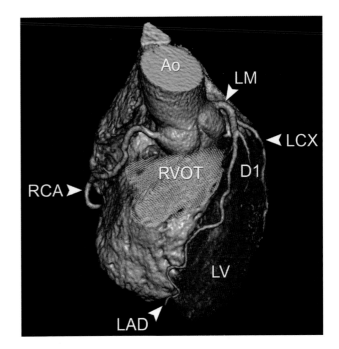

Figure 3.1 Volume-rendered image: superior anterior view of left and right coronary arteries. Ao, aorta; LM, left main coronary artery; LAD, left anterior descending; LCX, left circumflex coronary artery; RCA, right coronary artery; RVOT, right ventricular outflow tract; D1, first diagonal branch

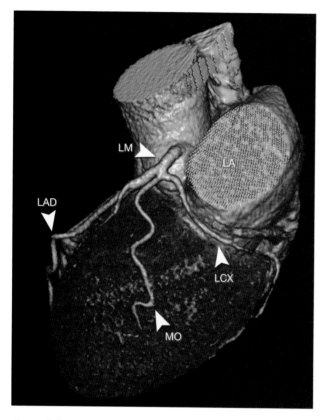

Figure 3.2 Volume-rendered image: lateral left view of left coronary artery. LM, left main coronary artery; LAD, left anterior descending artery; MO, marginal obtuse branch; LCX, left circumflex artery; LA, left atrium

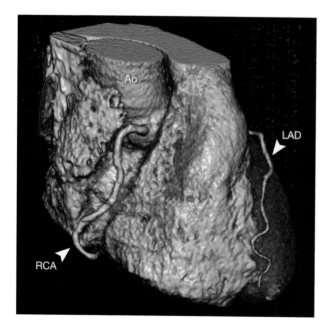

Figure 3.3 Volume-rendered image: lateral right view of right coronary artery (RCA). Ao, aorta; LAD, left anterior descending artery

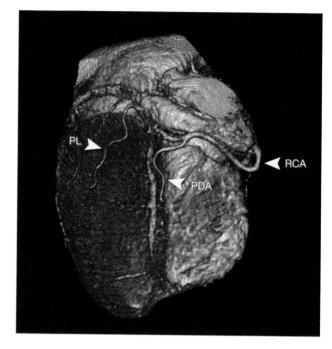

Figure 3.4 Volume-rendered image: inferior view of right coronary artery (RCA). PL, posterolateral branch; PDA, posterior descending artery

point where the atrioventricular groove and the posterior interventricular groove meet (Figures 3.3 and 3.4). In the majority (80%) of individuals the RCA is the dominant vessel and continues forwards from the crux along the posterior interventricular groove to become the posterior descending artery (PDA) (Figures 3.5 and 3.6). The posterolateral branch supplying the postero-inferior aspect of the left ventricle also arises from the RCA close to the crux. Left coronary dominance exists when the PDA arises from the circumflex artery (Figures 3.7 and 3.8). A balanced situation exists when the RCA and left circumflex (LCX) are of similar size.

The tomographic axial slices (the source slices) are normally used to visualize the coronary arteries. The course of the coronary arteries on the axial slices in relation to other cardiac structures is presented at different levels of the heart, as shown in Figures 3. 9 and 3.10.

CONCLUSION

The coronary anatomy can easily be assessed from the volume-rendered CT cardiac images. Knowledge of the gross anatomy of the coronary arteries is essential for accurate CT image interpretation.

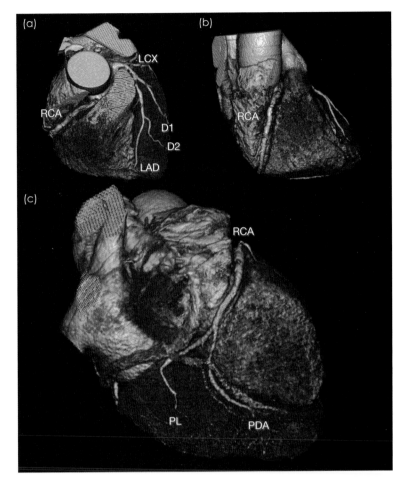

Figure 3.5 (a) Volume-rendered image: superior view of right and left coronary arteries. Left anterior descending (LAD) gives rise to two large diagonal branches. (b) Volume-rendered image of right coronary artery (RCA). (c) Volume-rendered image: inferior view of right dominant coronary artery. D1, first diagonal; D2, second diagonal; LCX, left circumflex; PL, posterolateral branch; PDA, posterior descending artery

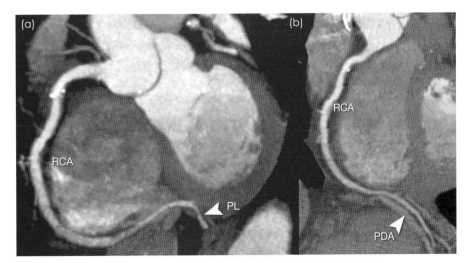

Figure 3.6 Same patient as in Figure 3.5. (a) Maximum-intensity projection of right coronary artery (RCA) and posterolateral branch (PL). (b) Curved multiplanar reconstruction of RCA and posterior descending artery (PDA)

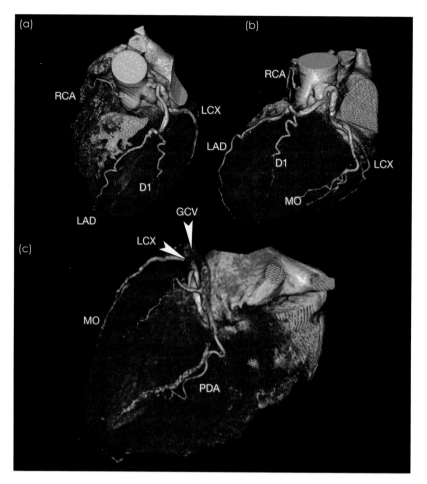

Figure 3.7 (a) Volume-rendered image: superior anterior view of left circumflex (LCX). (b) Volume-rendered image: lateral left view of left circumflex. (c) Volume-rendered image: inferior view of dominant left circumflex. Note: GCV obscures the course of LCX. RCA, right coronary artery; LAD, left anterior descending artery; D1, first diagonal branch; GCV, great cardiac vein; MO, marginal obtuse branch; PDA, posterior descending artery

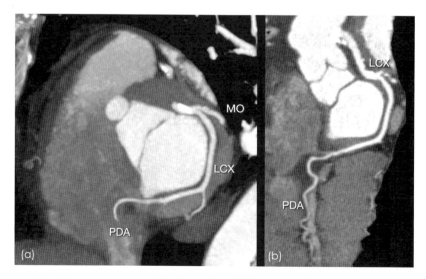

Figure 3.8 (a) Maximum-intensity projection of left circumflex (LCX) running in the atrioventricular groove. (b) Curved multiplanar reconstruction of the left circumflex. MO, marginal obtuse branch; PDA, posterior descending artery

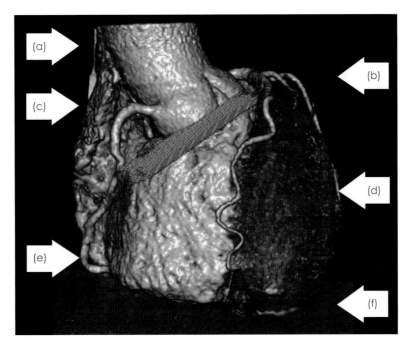

Figure 3.9 Volume-rendered image of coronary arteries. The arrows indicate the levels of the heart where axial images of the coronary arteries are chosen and shown in Figure 3.10

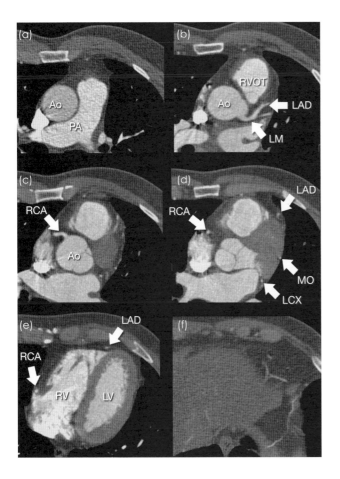

Figure 3.10 Axial images of coronary arteries at different levels of the heart. (a)–(f) From the base to the apex of the heart. (a) Level at aortic root and common pulmonary artery (PA). (b) Level at origin of left coronary artery. (c) Level at origin of right coronary artery (RCA). (d) Level of right coronary artery and left circumflex (LCX) at atrioventricular groove. (e) Mid-ventricular level: RCA. (f) Dome of the diaphragm. Ao, aorta; RVOT, right ventricular outflow tract; LM, left main; LAD, left anterior descending; MO, marginal obtuse branch; RV, right ventricle; LV, left ventricle

BIBLIOGRAPHY

Braunwald E. Heart disease. A Textbook of Cardiovascular Medicine, 4th edn. Philadelphia: W.B. Saunders,1992

James T. Anatomy of the coronary arteries in health and disease. Circulation 1965; 32: 1020–33

Levin DC, Harrington DP, Bettmann MA, et al. Anatomic variations of the coronary arteries supplying the anterolateral aspect of the left ventricle; possible explanation for the 'unexplained' anterior aneurysms. Invest Radiol 1982; 17: 458–62

Yamanaka O, Hobbs R. Coronary artery anomalies in 126 595 patients undergoing coronary angiography. Cathet Cardiovasc Diagn 1990; 21: 28–40

CHAPTER 4

Coronary pathology relevant to coronary imaging

A thorough review of the pathogenesis of coronary atherosclerosis is beyond the scope of this book; however, we believe it is worthwhile to provide a simple framework of the pathogenesis of coronary atherosclerosis to facilitate better understanding and interpretation of coronary plaque images.

The natural history of lumen atherosclerotic disease from the initial, only microscopically visible, lipid-filled macrophages to advanced lesions, that cause symptoms, is represented in the morphological classification scheme for lesions proposed by the American Heart Association (AHA)[1,2] (Table 4.1).

This classification scheme has been widely accepted as the framework of our current understanding of the progression of atherosclerosis. However, this scheme emphasizes mainly the histological features of plaque progression. From a clinical point of view, one might be more interested in a classification of coronary plaques that are associated with pathogenetic mechanisms associated with intracoronary thrombus formation and subsequent occurrence of acute coronary syndromes or sudden cardiac death.

Davies *et al.* demonstrated that rupture of the fibrous cap of an advanced atherosclerotic plaque exposes thrombogenic plaque components, in particular, tissue factor, to circulating blood thereby initiating platelet aggregation and intracoronary thrombus formation[3–5]. The fibrous cap is the region of the plaque that separates the necrotic core from the lumen, and when the thickness of the cap is less than 65 µm it may be vulnerable to rupture. Typically, ruptured lesions have a large necrotic, lipid core with a disrupted fibrous cap infiltrated by macrophages and lymphocytes and very small number of smooth muscle cells (Figure 4.1). Plaque rupture is the most common cause of acute coronary thrombosis formation and occurs in approximately 65–70% of cases. However, another cause of coronary thrombosis is plaque erosion[7,8]. Erosion occurs much less frequently, in approximately 25–30% of cases, and in these lesions, typically, the endothelium is absent at the erosion site.

Table 4.1 Current American Heart Association classification[1,2]

Type	Histological classification	Gross classification	Lesion	MSCT detection
I	isolated macrophage foam cells	fatty dot, fatty streak	early lesion	no
II	multiple foam cell layers	fatty dot, fatty streak	minimal lesion	no
III	preatheroma		intermediate	?
IV	atheroma	fibrolipid plaque	advanced	yes
V	fibroatheroma	fibrous plaque, plaque	advanced	yes
VI	fissured, ulcerated, hemorrhagic, thrombotic lesion	complicated lesion	advanced	yes
VII	calcific lesion	calcified lesion	advanced	yes
VIII	fibrotic lesion		advanced	yes

These lesions usually do not have a necrotic core, but if present this is small; they have a thick fibrous cap, and smooth muscle cells and proteoglycans are abundant while the eroded site contains minimal inflammation[7,8] (Figure 4.2). The majority of plaque erosions are eccentric and occur most frequently in young men and women < 50 years of age, often associated with smoking. Finally, a calcified nodule, albeit infrequent (2–5%), may be the cause of a thrombotic occlusion. Calcific nodules are plaques with luminal thrombi showing a calcific nodule protruding into the lumen through a disrupted thin fibrous cap[8] (Figure 4.2b). This plaque is associated with a large underlying calcific plaque. The lesion is usually seen in elderly male patients with heavily calcified and tortuous arteries.

Based on our recent knowledge that intracoronary thrombosis formation is caused by plaque rupture, plaque erosion and calcific nodule, which are associated with certain types of coronary plaques, Virmani et al. proposed a modified AHA lesion classification[8] (Table 4.2). This modified AHA lesion classification describes the progression of atherosclerotic lesions from early stages through to advanced thrombosis-prone plaques. It forms an important link between histology, intracoronary thrombus formation and clinical presentation of coronary artery disease. The classification may further

guide evolving research into the identification of a high-risk (vulnerable) plaque.

For the purpose of multislice CT (MSCT) plaque imaging we have adapted and simplified this modified AHA classification (Table 4.2)[8].

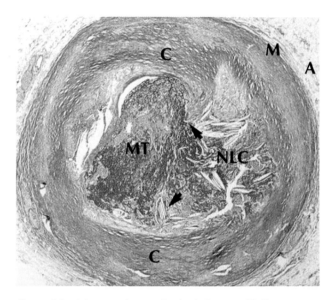

Figure 4.1 Advanced complicated plaque with fibrous cap rupture. MT, mural thrombus; NLC, necrotic lipid core; C, collagen; M, media; A, adventitia; arrow, rupture fibrous cap. From reference 6, with permission

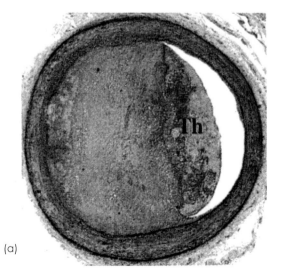

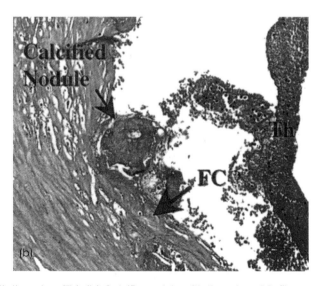

Figure 4.2 Plaque erosion/calcific nodule. (a) Plaque erosion with thrombus (Th). (b) Calcific nodule with thrombus. FC, fibrous cap. From reference 8, with permission

Table 4.2 Modified American Heart Association classification based on morphological description of progressive atherosclerotic lesions. From reference 8, with permission

Figures	Fibrous cap atheroma	Necrotic core with overlying fibrous cap
4.1	Thin fibrous cap atheroma	thin fibrous cap, infiltrated by macrophages and lymphocytes with rare smooth muscle cells and an underlying necrotic core
4.2b	Calcified nodule	rupture of nodular calcification with underlying fibrocalcific plaque
4.3	Fibrocalcific plaque	collagen-rich plaque with significant stenosis usually contains large areas of calcification with few inflammatory cells
4.1 & 4.2a	Intracoronary thrombosis	erosion or rupture causing non-occlusive or occlusive thrombus

IN VIVO MSCT CORONARY PLAQUE IMAGING

The current resolution of MSCT scanners does not permit the initial phases of coronary atherosclerosis to be identified, and it cannot distinguish between plaque rupture and erosion as the cause of intracoronary thrombosis. Furthermore, the more subtle features of a plaque, such as fibrous cap thickness, disruption or signs of inflammation, cannot be seen. Because of its limited resolution non-invasive MSCT only allows the depiction of advanced lesions according to the AHA classification or progressive atherosclerotic lesions according to the modified AHA classification. Advanced plaques may or may not be associated with lumenal narrowing depending on the presence of compensatory vessel wall remodeling that tends to preserve the lumen size in the earlier stages of plaque progression. CT coronary plaque imaging allows plaques to be classified as obstructive or non-obstructive. However, to date, precise quantification of the size of plaques is not possible either due to over- or underestimation and lack of quantification algorithms. In general, the size of low-density plaques tends to be underestimated and the size of calcific plaques tends to be overestimated. The precise composition of tissues within the plaque cannot be accurately assessed. MSCT can easily discriminate between a low- and high-density plaque. Low-density plaques represent either lipid core, necrotic or fibrous tissue and high-density plaques represent calcium, whereas in the setting of an acute coronary syndrome a very low-density lesion of the culprit artery may be assumed to be a thrombotic lesion.

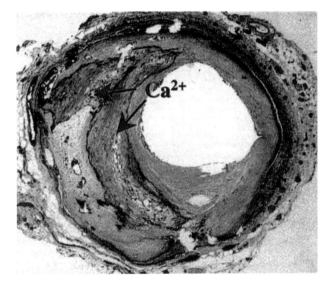

Figure 4.3 Fibrocalcific plaque. Ca^{2+}: calcium. From reference 8 with permission

Current MSCT scanners cannot reliably discriminate between lipid accumulation in the plaque and fibrous tissue, and, to date, cannot reliably identify a plaque prone to rupture. Higher-resolution scanners may resolve this problem.

CONCLUSION

MSCT plaque imaging allows, albeit rather crudely, discrimination between different types of advanced coronary plaques (Table 4.3 and Figures 4.4–4.9).

Table 4.3 MSCT features helpful to identify plaques

Figure	MSCT features	Density (HU)	Advanced plaques (AHA)	Progressive atherosclerotic lesion (modified AHA)
4.4	high density	> 150	—	calcific nodule
4.5	high density	> 150	calcific plaque	—
4.6	high–low density		—	fibrocalcific plaque
4.7	intermediate density	50–100	fibrous plaque	fibrous cap atheroma
4.8	low density	20–50	(fibro)atheroma	thin fibrous cap atheroma
4.9	very low density	< 20	complicated plaque	thrombus

AHA, American Heart Association

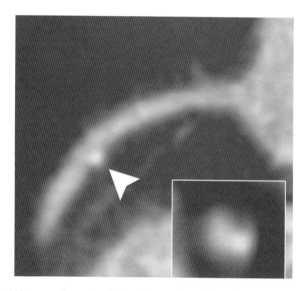

Figure 4.4 Axial and cross-sectional image of small calcific plaque (arrowhead small high-density plaque (375 HU))

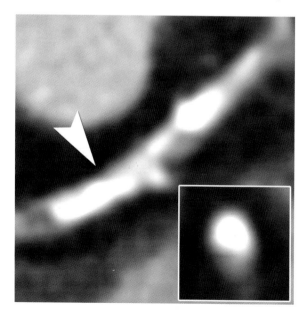

Figure 4.5 Axial and cross-sectional image of calcific plaque (arrowhead high-density plaque (480 HU))

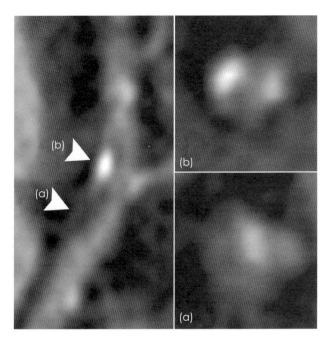

Figure 4.6 Axial and cross-sectional images of fibrocalcific plaque. (Arrowhead (a); low-density (40 HU) and arrowhead (b): high density (350 HU))

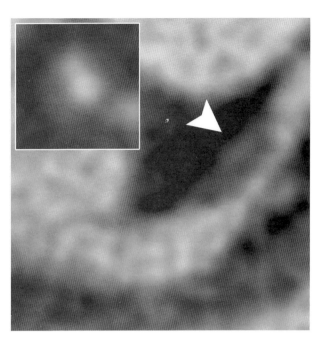

Figure 4.8 Axial and cross-sectional images of (fibro) lipid plaque. (Arrowhead: low-density plaque (35 HU))

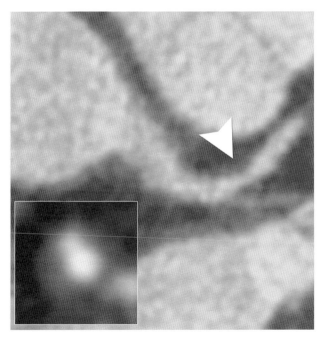

Figure 4.7 Axial and cross-sectional images of fibrotic plaque. (Arrowhead: intermediate-density plaque (95 HU))

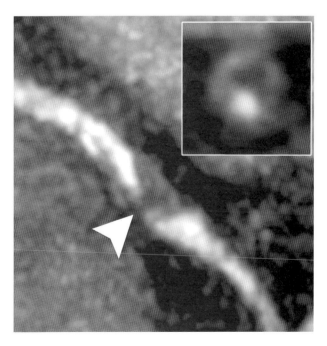

Figure 4.9 Axial and cross-sectional images of thrombotic occlusion. (Arrowhead: very low-density plaque (10 HU))

REFERENCES

1. Stary HC, Chandler AB, Glagov S, et al. A definition of initial, fatty streak, and intermediate lesions of atherosclerosis. A report from the Committee on Vascular Lesions of the Council on Arteriosclerosis, American Heart Association. Arterioscler Thromb 1994; 14: 840–56

2. Stary HC, Chandler AB, Dinsmore RE, et al. A definition of advanced types of atherosclerotic lesions and a histological classification of atherosclerosis. A report from the Committee on Vascular Lesions of the Council on Arteriosclerosis, American Heart Association. Arterioscler Thromb Vasc Biol 1995; 15: 1512–31

3. Davies MJ, Thomas AC. Plaque fissuring – the cause of acute myocardial infarction, sudden ischaemic death, and crescendo angina. Br Heart J 1985; 53: 363–73

4. Davies MJ. Anatomic features in victims of sudden coronary death. Coronary artery pathology. Circulation 1992; 85 (Suppl 1): I19–24

5. Falk E. Plaque rupture with severe pre-existing stenosis precipitating coronary thrombosis. Characteristics of coronary atherosclerotic plaques underlying fatal occlusive thrombi. Br Heart J 1983; 50: 127–34

6. Wilson PWF. Atlas of Atherosclerosis. Risk factors and Treatment, 3rd edn, Part 1. Philadelphia: Current Medicine, Inc

7. van der Wal AC, Becker AE, van der Loos CM, Das PK. Site of intimal rupture or erosion of thrombosed coronary atherosclerotic plaques is characterized by an inflammatory process irrespective of the dominant plaque morphology. Circulation 1994; 89: 36–44

8. Virmani R, Kolodgie FD, Burke AP, Farb A, Schwartz SM. Lessons from sudden coronary death: a comprehensive morphological classification scheme for atherosclerotic lesions. Arterioscler Thromb Vasc Biol 2000; 20: 1262–75

CHAPTER 5

Coronary stenosis

Conventional X-ray coronary angiography with selective contrast enhancement of the coronary arteries is still regarded as the reference standard for *in vivo* detection and quantification of coronary artery stenosis. High-resolution projections of only the contrast-enhanced coronary arteries are acquired at a high frame rate throughout the cardiac cycle. It provides accurate lesion depiction and quantification of the stenosis severity. The flow of contrast through the vessel gives an impression of the coronary flow. Finally, catheter-based angiography can be complemented with advanced coronary imaging techniques, such as intracoronary ultrasound (ICUS) or optical coherence tomography (OCT), and flow or pressure measurements to determine the functional severity of a coronary obstruction. While it seems unlikely that a non-invasive technique such as multislice computed tomography (MSCT) can ever replace invasive coronary angiography, there may be situations where sufficient information regarding the coronary integrity may be acquired by a non-invasive technique with benefits in terms of cost, patient risk and discomfort.

IMAGING CHARACTERISTICS

MSCT coronary angiograms are different from conventional angiograms. Conventional angiograms are projections of a vessel that has been enhanced with a high concentration of contrast material (Figure 5.1). During the injection of contrast, multiple images of this vessel are acquired throughout a number of cycles. For MSCT angiography the cross-sectional images of the coronary arteries are reconstructed during a single phase of a number of consecutive heart cycles (Figure 5.1). Because contrast is injected intravenously and scanning is per-

formed during the plateau phase of the contrast enhancement, all blood-containing cavities are opacified. The intracoronary blood opacification in MSCT is of a relatively low magnitude and calcium or stents having high densities are much more visible, compared to conventional angiography (Figure 5.2). The technical boundaries of CT limit the spatial and temporal resolution, which are significantly lower than in catheter-based angiography (Table 5.1). This limits the applicability of stenosis severity quantification software, particularly in the smaller branches. On the other hand, because MSCT is a cross-sectional technique, it allows appreciation of the non-enhanced soft tissues in the proximity of the vessels and allows for three-dimensional reconstruction of the cardiac and coronary anatomy (Figure 5.3).

DIAGNOSTIC PERFORMANCE

The diagnostic performance of electron-beam (EB)CT[1–10], four-slice MSCT[11–19], eight-slice MSCT[20] and 16-slice MSCT[21–24] for the detection of significant coronary stenosis, as reported in a number of comparative studies with conventional angiography, can be found in Tables 5.2–5.4 (Figures 5.4–5.6). These studies were performed with comparable equipment but varied in study design, i.e. patient population, scan protocols and data analysis. In all studies the patient population consisted of individuals with anginal symptoms and a high disease prevalence: between 0.9 and 1.6 lesions or significantly diseased vessels per patient. Some studies evaluated each coronary segment separately, while others evaluated the entire coronary artery as a single entity. Either a specific number of proximal, middle and distal segments, or all coronary segments with a

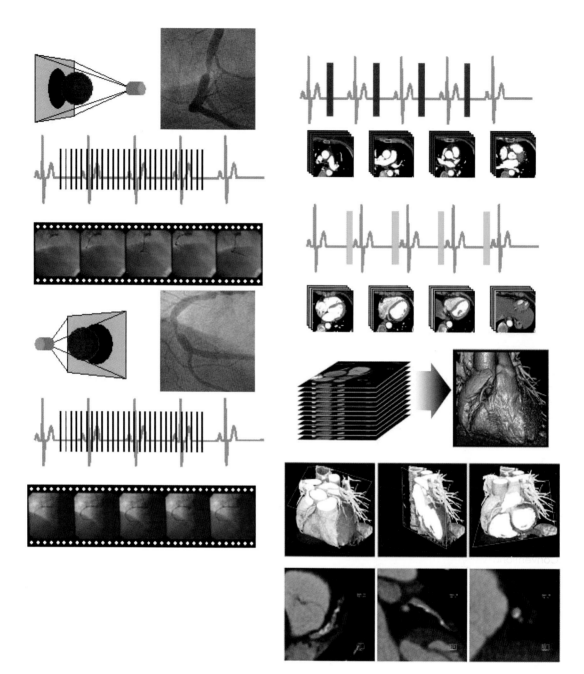

Figure 5.1 Coronary angiograms (CAG) versus multislice CT (MSCT) coronary imaging. While contrast is selectively injected into the coronary artery, more than 20 roentgen projections are acquired, showing the dynamic contrast enhancement of the vessel. Computer-assisted contour-detected quantification of a coronary stenosis (minimum lumen diameter) requires at least two perpendicular projections. The minimum lumenal diameter is calculated as the average of the shortest diameters in the two perpendicular projections. MSCT requires intravenous injection of contrast and data are acquired during the steady state of contrast enhancement. During each cycle a consecutive and overlapping volume of the heart is scanned. Images are reconstructed during mid-diastolic phase in the heart cycle and reconstruction of an entire volume requires isocardiophasic data from a sequence of heart cycles. Different phases can be reconstructed depending on the position of the reconstruction window within the R-to-R interval. From these individual slices a three-dimensional data volume can be created that allows reconstruction of cross-sectional planes through the volume and display of the vessel or lesion of interest at any position or angle. If the spatial resolution in relation to the vessel size permits, stenosis quantification can be performed by direct measurement of the vessel area

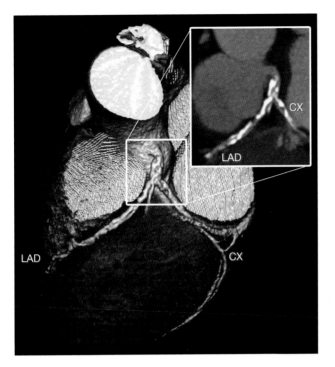

Figure 5.2 Volume-rendered (colored image) and maximum intensity projection (insert). CT images readily highlight the presence of coronary calcifications (high-density structures are displayed as white). CX, circumflex coronary artery; LAD, left anterior descending coronary artery

specified minimal lumen diameter, were included. Over time the use of beta-receptor blockers has become routine. In a study with 16-slice MSCT by Nieman *et al.* patients with a pre-scan heart rate over 65 bpm were given an oral dose of 100 mg metoprolol 1 h prior to the examination, resulting in an overall average heart rate of 57 bpm[21]. Ropers *et al.* used 50 mg of atenolol if the heart rate was more than 60 bpm, which resulted in an average heart rate of 62 bpm[22].

IMAGE INTERPRETABILITY (Table 5.5)

To determine whether a CT angiogram, or part of a CT angiogram, is evaluable or not depends on a number of factors, including observer experience and confidence. Using four-slice MSCT, the number of segments with a subjectively adequate image quality varied between 6% and 43% in the different studies (Table 5.3). Recent studies with 16-slice technology and routine beta-receptor blocking report that only between 6% and 12% of the coronary branches contained sections with poor image quality (Table 5.4)[21–24]. The main reasons for reduced assessability are related to motion artifacts caused by residual cardiac motion, severe coronary calci-

Table 5.1 Conventional versus MSCT coronary angiography

	Conventional angiography	*MSCT angiography*
Contrast injection	intracoronary	intravenous (peripheral)
Contrast enhancement	selective coronary	complete vascular
Image acquisition	projection	cross-section (3D)
Acquisition rate	~20 projections per heart cycle	1 data set in ~20 heart cycles
Radiation exposure	3–10 mSv	5–13 mSv
Examination time	≥1 h	<30 min
In-hospital time	≤1 day	1–2 h
Spatial resolution	0.1×0.1×∞ mm	0.7×0.7×0.7 mm
Temporal resolution	≤50 ms	(50–)200 ms
Additional advantages	lesion quantification coronary flow additional diagnostics (IVUS, pressure measurements, etc.) intervention	minimally invasive procedure cardiac anatomy plaque imaging
Additional disadvantages	complications and discomfort related to the arterial puncture and coronary intubation	sensitive to arrhythmia calcified vessels

IVUS, intravascular ultrasound; ∞, infinity

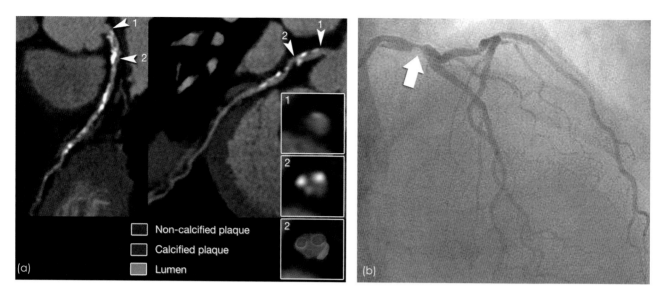

Figure 5.3 (a) Curved multiplanar reconstructed images of the left main and left anterior descending coronary arteries in two orthogonal directions (large images) showing a severely diseased left main coronary artery and the presence of both calcified and non-calcified tissue components. Cross-sectional images at different levels of the left main coronary artery (arrowheads) suggest significant narrowing of the coronary lumen. Arrowheads at site of cross-sectional images (1) and (2). At (2) narrow-lumen large mixed plaque and remodeling. (b) Invasive angiography confirming the presence of a significant stenosis in the left main coronary artery (arrow)

Table 5.2 Diagnostic performance of contrast-enhanced electron-beam computed tomography with conventional coronary angiography as the standard of reference

	Patients	Sensitivity (%)	Specificity (%)	Excluded (%)
Moshage et al.[1]	20	74	100	NR
Achenbach et al.[2]	125	92	94	25
Rensing et al.[3]	37	77	94	19
Reddy et al.[4]	23	88	79	8
Schmermund et al.[5]	28	83	91	12
Nakanishi et al.[6]	37	74	94	12
Budoff et al.[7]	52	78	91	11
Moshage et al.[8]	118	90	82	24
Achenbach et al.[9]	36	92	91	20
Lu et al.[10]	107	91	93	7

NR, not reported

fication and voluntary patient movement, but also include the occasional inability to discriminate the coronary artery lumen from adjacent contrast-enhanced structures, technical scanner failure and insufficient scan range (Table 5.5). With four-slice MSCT scanners a complete cardiac scan requires up to 40 s, which is too long for certain patients. During the long breath hold,

as well as injection of contrast medium, most patients experience an acceleration of the heart rate during the acquisition (Figure 5.7). Other incidental causes for reduced interpretability are motion and beam-hardening artifacts from the inflow of highly concentrated contrast medium in the superior caval vein or high-density artifacts from pacemaker wires. Patients with arrhyth-

Table 5.3 Diagnostic performance of four- and eight-slice MSCT to detect coronary stenosis, with conventional angiography as the standard of reference (four-slice CT)

	CT	Use of beta-blockers	(n)	Basis of assessment	Significant diameter reduction (%)	Previous disease per patient* (n)	Excluded segments or branches (%)	Sensitivity (%)	Specificity (%)	PPV (%)	NPV (%)	Sensitivity† (%)
Nieman et al.[11]	4	−	31	branch	50	0.9	27	81	97	81	97	68
Achenbach et al.[12]	4	−	64	branch	50 70	1.1 0.9	32 32	85 91	76 84	56 59	93 98	55 58
Knez et al.[13]	4	−	43	segment	50	1.2	6	78	98	84	96	51
Vogl et al.[14]	4	+	64	segment	50	NR	28	75	99	92	98	NR
Nieman et al.[15]	4	−	53	segment	50	1.3	30	82	93	66	97	61
Kopp et al.‡[16]	4	−	102	segment	50	1.5	15	86 93	96 97	76 81	98 99	86 93
Giesler et al.**[17]	4	+	100	branch	70	1.0	29	91	89	66	98	49
Nieman et al.**[18]	4	−	78	segment	50	0.9	32	84	95	67	98	63
Kuettner et al.[19]	4	+	66	segment	70	1.6	43	66	98	83	95	37
Maruyama et al.[20]	8	−	25	segment	50	1.5	14	90	99	93	99	73

*Number of diseased vessels or segments per patient; †overall sensitivity including missed lesions in non-assessable segments or branches; **studies that include patients from earlier publications; PPV, positive predictive value; and NPV, negative predictive value, with respect to the assessable segments and branches; NR, not reported

Table 5.4 Diagnostic performance of MSCT to detect coronary stenosis, with conventional angiography as the standard of reference (16-slice CT)

	CT	Use of beta-blockers	(n)	Basis of assessment	Significant diameter reduction (%)	Previous disease per patient* (n)	Excluded segments or branches (%)	Sensitivity (%)	Specificity (%)	PPV (%)	NPV (%)	Sensitivity† (%)
Nieman et al.[21]	12	+	58	> 2.0-mm branches	50	1.1	—	95	86	80	97	93
Ropers et al.[22]	12	+	77	> 1.5-mm branches	50	1.0	12	92	93	79	97	73
Kuettner et al.[23]	16	+	60	segments	50	1.2	6	72	97	72	97	NR
Mollet et al.[24]	16	+	128	segments	50	1.6	—	92	95	79	98	92

*Number of stenosed vessels or segments per patient; †overall sensitivity including missed lesions in non-assessable segments or branches; PPV, positive predictive value; and NPV, negative predictive value, regarding the assessable segments or branches; NR, not reported

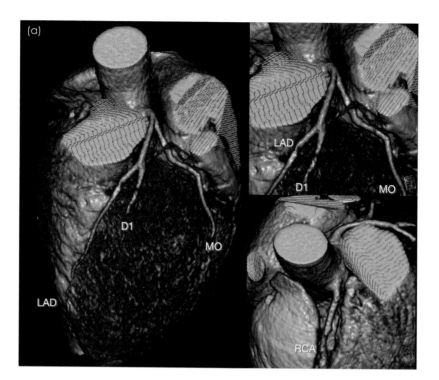

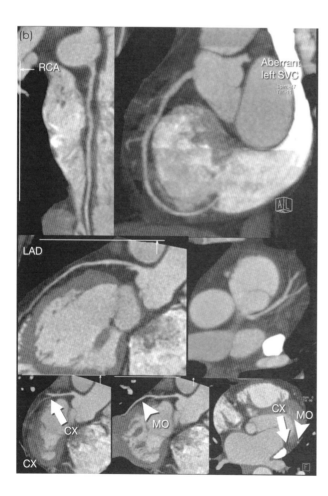

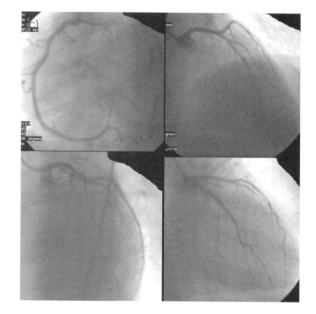

Figure 5.4 (a) Volume-rendered images of the main coronary arteries. No significant stenosis can be visualized. (b) Curved multiplanar reconstructed and maximum-intensity projected CT images of the same patient again do not show significant lumen narrowing of the main coronary arteries. An incidental finding is the presence of an aberrant left superior vena cava (SVC). (c) Invasive coronary angiography confirming absence of coronary stenosis. D1, first diagonal branch; LAD, left anterior descending coronary artery; MO, marginal obtuse branch; CX, circumflex coronary artery; RCA, right coronary artery

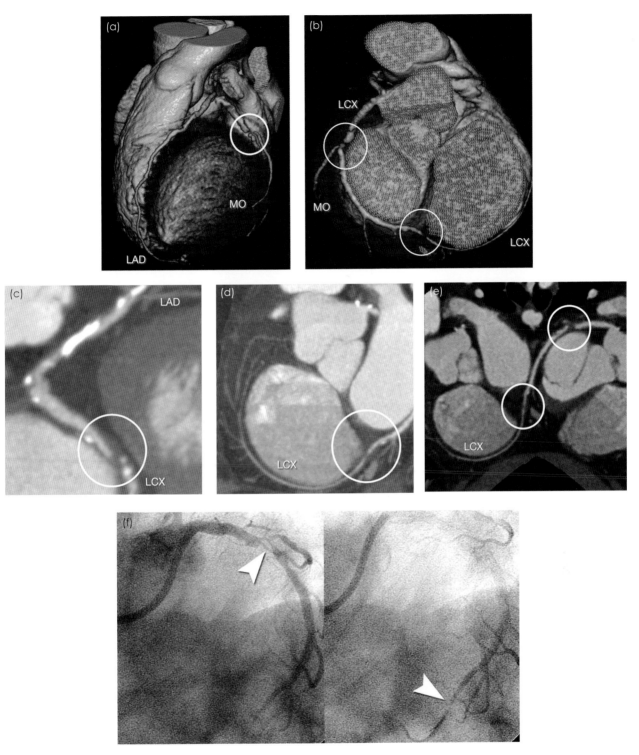

Figure 5.5 (a) Volume-rendered image (anterior view) showing a significant lesion (circle) located at the bifurcation of the circumflex coronary artery (LCX) and the first marginal obtuse branch (MO). (b) Volume-rendered image (posterior view) after removing the left and right atrium showing two significant lesions (circles). The proximal lesion is located at the bifurcation of the circumflex coronary artery and the first marginal obtuse branch, and the distal lesion in the posterolateral branch. Maximum-intensity projections of the proximal (c) and distal (d) coronary lesions. (e) Curved multiplanar reconstructed image of the circumflex coronary artery showing the proximal and distal coronary lesions. (f) Invasive angiography confirming the presence of both significant obstructive coronary lesions located in the circumflex coronary artery (arrowheads). LAD, left anterior descending coronary artery

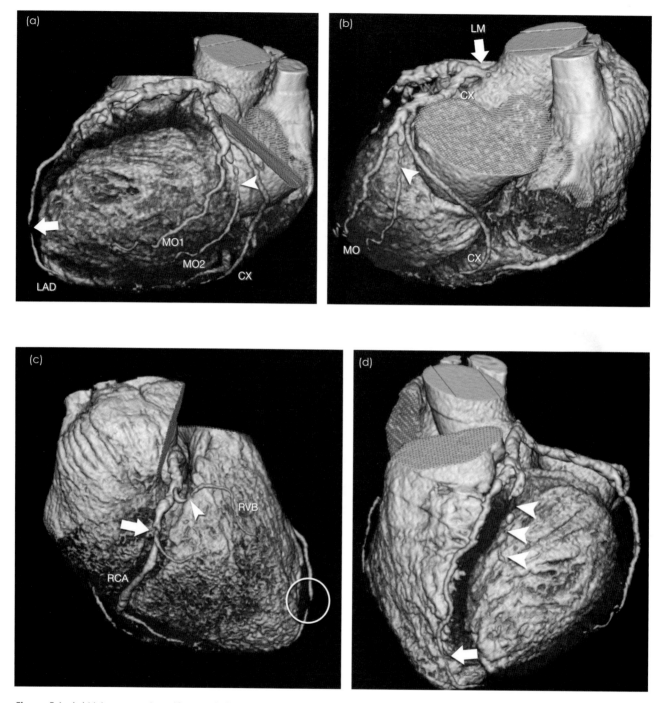

Figure 5.6 (a) Volume-rendered image (left lateral view) highlighting significant stenosis in the left anterior descending coronary artery (LAD) (arrow) and second marginal obtuse branch (MO2) (arrowhead). (b) Volume-rendered image (left posterolateral view) highlighting the significant stenosis in the second marginal obtuse branch (MO) (arrowhead). (c) Volume-rendered image (right posterolateral view) highlighting significant stenosis in the right coronary artery (RCA, arrow), right ventricular branch (RVB, arrowhead) and left anterior descending coronary artery (circle). (d) Volume-rendered image (anterior view) highlighting a total occlusion of the first diagonal branch (arrowheads) and a significant stenosis in the left anterior descending coronary artery (arrow). (e) Curved multiplanar reconstructed image of the left main and left anterior descending coronary artery, again showing the occluded first diagonal branch (box) and a significant lesion in the left anterior descending (arrow). The maximum-intensity projection (upper panel) and cross-sectional images (lower panels) visualize different plaque tissue components. (f) Curved multiplanar reconstructed images of the left circumflex (LCX) and right (RCA) coronary artery showing two significant lesions (arrows). (g) Invasive angiography confirming the presence of three-vessel disease (arrows, total occlusion of the first diagonal branch; arrowheads, significant stenoses). CX, circumflex coronary artery; MO1, first marginal obtuse branch

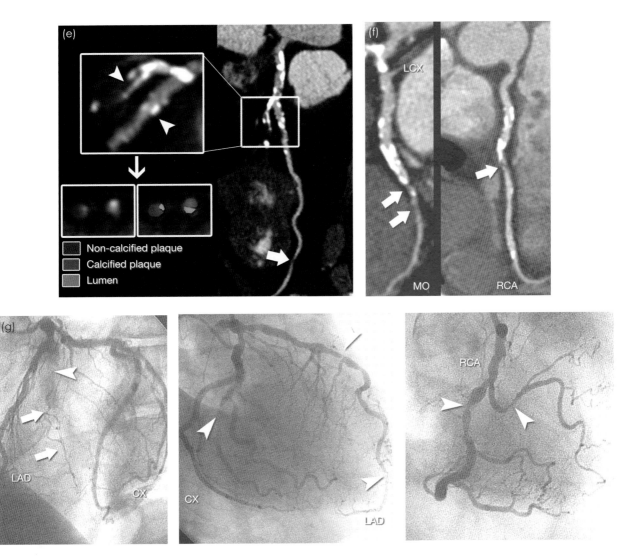

Figure 5.6 *Continued*

Table 5.5 Vessel image interpretability (%) for four-, eight- and 16-slice MSCT

	n	Analysis	RCA	LM	LAD	LCX	All
Four-slice MSCT							
Nieman et al.[11]	31	segments	71	97	86	52	73
Knez et al.[13]	44	segments	88	100	95	91	94
Vogl et al.[14]	64	segments 1–15	83	100	91	65	81
Nieman et al.[15]	53	>2.0-mm segments	67	98	77	53	70
Kopp et al.[16]	102	segments	70	100	87	90	85
Giesler et al.[17]	100	branches	52	92	76	65	71
Kuettner et al.	66	segments		97			57
Eight-slice MSCT							
Maruyama et al.[20]	25	>2.0-mm segments	91	100	91	66	86
16-slice MSCT							
Nieman et al.[21]	58	>2.0-mm branches	88	98	92	93	93

RCA, right coronary artery; LM, left main coronary artery; LAD, left anterior descending coronary artery; LCX, left circumflex coronary artery

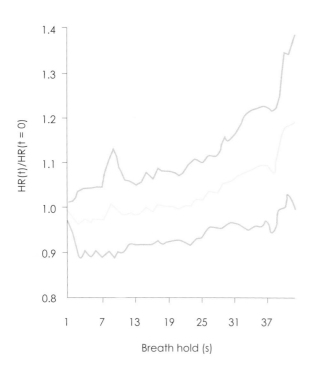

Figure 5.7 Averaged heart rate acceleration (yellow line) of ten patients during CT data acquisition. Green lines, range

Table 5.6 Factors influencing the image interpretability

Fixed scanner criteria
Temporal resolution
Spatial resolution
Contrast-to-noise

Fixed patient criteria
Arrhythmia
Patient size
Coronary size
Coronary calcification
Ability to hold breath
Metal objects: stents, pacemaker wires, etc.

Modifiable criteria
Contrast-enhancement protocol
Heart rate
Scan protocol: collimation, tube output
ECG gating
Patient population
Patient anxiety

Investigator related criteria
Experience
Confidence

mia are generally denied MSCT coronary angiography because of the beat-to-beat end-diastolic volume variation. However, occasional premature contractions, which occur in many patients, can also adversely affect the assessment. The contrast enhancement also influences the interpretability, and when stenosis detection of lumenal narrowing is the objective, a high intracoronary concentration of contrast media is preferred. Finally, patient size adversely affects the quality of the scan (Table 5.6).

In all published studies, the left main coronary artery could be evaluated in the vast majority of cases (Table 5.5) (Figure 5.8). The left anterior descending coronary artery (LAD) may suffer from extensive calcification but is less frequently affected by motion artifacts (Figure 5.9). Severe calcification may compromise identification of stenosis. The right coronary artery (RCA), which has a large motion radius and short motion-sparse period during diastole, is more susceptible to motion artifacts, caused by residual cardiac motion during the image reconstruction interval (Figure 5.10). The left circumflex coronary artery (LCX) also suffers from motion artifacts. Particularly, when scanning continues late after

contrast injection, venous structures may be enhanced and thereby more difficult to discriminate from for instance the LCX. In a four-slice MSCT study comparing the assessability of the different coronary segments with a minimal diameter of 2.0 mm, the proximal RCA was evaluable in 88%, compared to 61% of the middle and 60% of the distal segments, while assessment of the proximal LAD was possible in 89%, compared to 77% of the middle and 75% of the distal segments. In this study the proximal and middle segments of the LCX were equally difficult to evaluate, 57% and 56%, respectively[15].

STENOSIS DETECTION

If only coronary arteries or segments with sufficient image quality are considered, the sensitivity of four-slice MSCT to detect ≥ 50% coronary obstruction ranges between 66% and 95%, and the specificity between 76% and 99% (Table 5.3), with an inverse correlation between the sensitivity and specificity. There is also an inverse relationship between the diagnostic performance

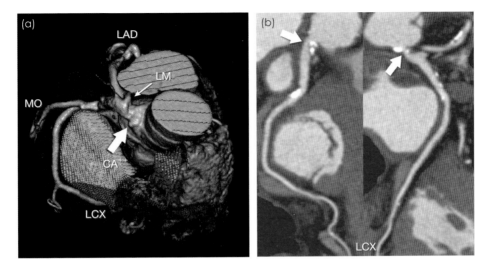

Figure 5.8 (a) Volume-rendered image (left posterolateral view) showing severe calcification of the left main coronary artery (LM). The calcified plaque completely obscures the presence of a significant lumen narrowing of the left main coronary artery. (b) Curved multiplanar reconstructions of the left main and left circumflex coronary artery (LCX) in two orthogonal directions show a significant stenosis of the left main (arrows). Ca++, calcium plaque; LAD, left anterior descending coronary artery; MO, marginal obtuse branch

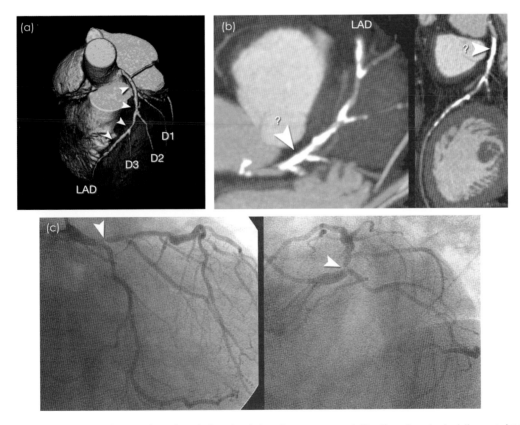

Figure 5.9 (a) Volume-rendered image (cranioanterior view) showing severe calcifications located at the proximal and mid-part of the left anterior descending coronary artery (LAD). (b) Maximum-intensity projection (left panel) and curved multiplanar reconstructed image (right panel) of the left anterior descending coronary artery. In this case, the presence of severe calcifications completely obscures the coronary lumen, which precludes evaluation of the proximal and mid-part of the left anterior descending coronary artery. (c, d) Invasive angiography showing a significant lesion located at the proximal left anterior descending coronary artery (arrowheads). This lesion was evidently missed on the MSCT coronary angiogram owing to severe calcifications. D1, first diagonal branch; D2, second diagonal branch; D3, third diagonal branch

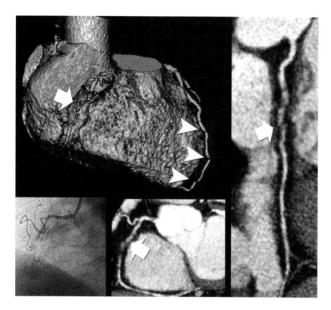

Figure 5.10 An occluded right coronary artery (arrows) with collateral filling is visualized using different post-processing techniques. This finding was confirmed with invasive coronary angiography (left lower panel). However, image quality of the MSCT angiogram is severely reduced due to the motion artifacts. These motion artifacts affected not only the evaluation of the right coronary artery, but also the evaluation of the left anterior descending coronary artery (arrowheads)

and the number of assessable segments. The diagnostic performance is obviously better in segments with a larger lumen diameter[15]. The segments and vessels that were excluded from analysis because of inadequate image quality contained a substantial number of undetected lesions. If these lesions in non-evaluable vessels are included in the analysis, as false-negative interpretations, the sensitivity is much lower in most studies, between 37% and 93% (Tables 5.3–5.5).

To date, four studies have been published that compare MSCT and conventional coronary angiography using 16-slice MSCT (Table 5.4)[21–24]. Nieman et al., irrespectively of the image quality, evaluated all branches with a minimal lumenal diameter of 2.0 mm, and found a sensitivity and specificity of 95% and 86%, respectively, to detect significantly stenosed branches. The positive and negative predictive values were reported as 80% and 97%, respectively[21]. All four missed lesions were located in the left circumflex coronary artery and obtuse marginal branches, no lesions were missed in the left main, left anterior descending or right coronary artery. Including only the evaluable (88%) vessels (minimal diameter of 1.5 mm), Ropers et al. found a sensitivity and specificity of 92% and 93%,

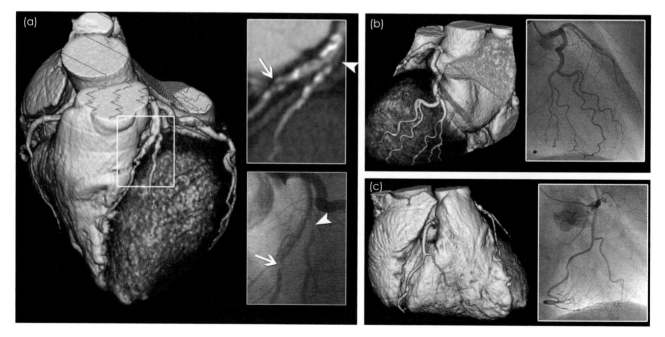

Figure 5.11 (a) Volume-rendered image (anterior view) providing an anatomical overview of the left coronary artery. Detail: maximum-intensity projection showing a significant lesion of the mid-part of the left anterior descending coronary artery and an ostial lesion of the first diagonal branch. Both lesions were confirmed on the conventional angiogram (right lower panel). (b) Volume-rendered image (left lateral view) and corresponding conventional angiogram of the circumflex coronary artery. No significant lesions are visualized. (c) Volume-rendered image (right lateral view) and corresponding invasive angiogram of the right coronary artery. No significant lesions are visualized

respectively, to detect significant stenoses. Without exclusion of non-evaluable lesions the sensitivity was 73%[22]. Kuettner *et al.* investigated 60 patients with 16-slice MSCT. After exclusion of 6% of the coronary segments from analysis due to poor image quality, they detected significant stenoses (> 50% diameter reduction) with a sensitivity of 72% and specificity of 97%[23].

Mollet *et al.* investigated a total of 128 patients with a sensitivity and specificity to detect significant lesions of 92% and 93%, respectively (Figures 5.11 and 5.12)[24].

In our opinion MSCT of the coronary arteries allows only limited quantification of the stenosis severity, but generally more severe lesions, according to catheter angiography, are detected with a higher sensitivity[12].

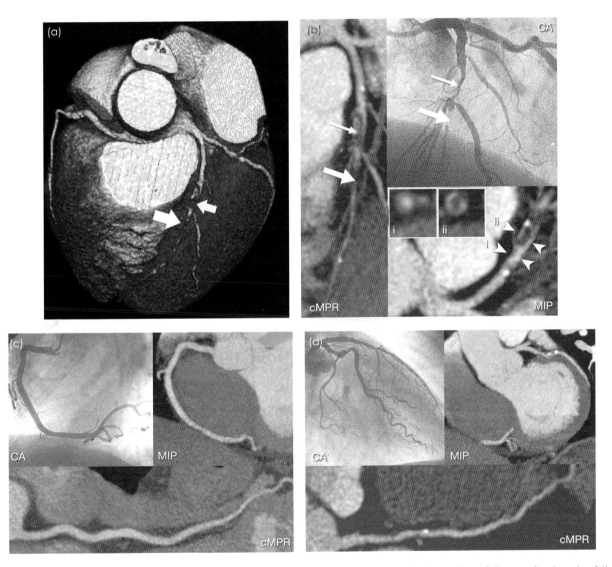

Figure 5.12 (a) Volume-rendered image (cranioanterior view) showing an anatomical overview of the proximal parts of the main coronary arteries. A significant lesion of the mid-part (small arrow) and a total occlusion of the distal part (large arrow) of the left anterior descending coronary artery are visualized. (b) Different post-processing techniques (curved multiplanar reconstruction (cMPR) and maximum intensity projection (MIP)) are used to visualize the coronary lesions in more detail (arrows). Cross-sectional images (i) and (ii) at different locations (arrowheads) illustrate a high-grade stenosis of the mid-part of the left anterior descending coronary artery and calcified as well as non-calcified plaque tissue components. Both lesions were confirmed on invasive coronary angiogram (CA). (c) Maximum-intensity projection and curved multiplanar reconstruction CT images of the right coronary artery rule out the presence of significant lesions. These findings are confirmed on the corresponding invasive coronary angiogram. (d) Maximum-intensity projection and curved multiplanar reconstruction CT images of the circumflex coronary artery rule out the presence of significant lesions. These findings are confirmed on the corresponding invasive coronary angiogram

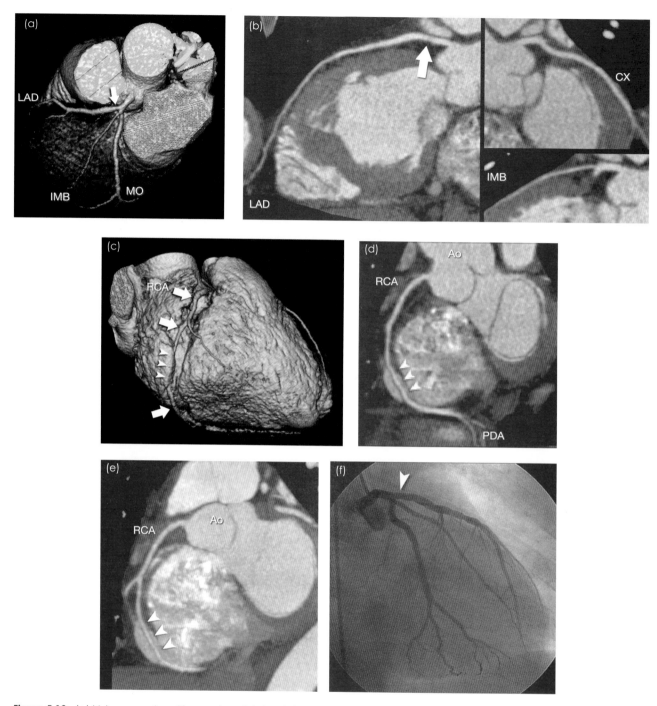

Figure 5.13 (a) Volume-rendered image (craniolateral view) providing an anatomical overview of the left coronary artery. This image suggests a non-significant lesion (arrow) located at the proximal part of the left anterior descending coronary artery (LAD). (b) The presence of a non-significant lesion located at the proximal part of the left anterior descending coronary artery is also visualized on multiplanar reconstructed images. No significant lesions are visualized throughout the left coronary system. (c) Volume-rendered image (right lateral view) providing an anatomical overview of the right coronary artery (RCA). An incidental finding is the aberrant course of the RCA running within the right atrium (arrowheads). (d) Curved multiplanar reconstruction of the right coronary artery ruling out significant stenoses. The aberrant course of the RCA is again visualized (arrowheads). (e) Maximum-intensity projection confirming the findings of the other image processing techniques. Arrowheads indicate the aberrant course of the right coronary artery. (f) Invasive angiography image confirming the presence of only a non-significant lesion (arrowhead) within the left coronary artery. IMB, intermediate coronary branch; MO, marginal obtuse coronary branch; CX, circumflex coronary artery; IMB, intermediate coronary branch; Ao, aorta; PDA, posterior descending coronary artery

Table 5.7 Patient-based diagnostic performance of MSCT coronary angiography

	Four-slice MSCT segment-based analysis in 53 patients[15]				16-slice MSCT vessel-based analysis in 58 patients[21]			
	Accuracy		Predictive value		Accuracy		Predictive value	
	n	%	n	%	n	%	n	%
No significant lesion	(9/14)	64%	(9/19)	47%	(7/7)	100%	(7/8)	88%
Single lesion/vessel	(9/23)	39%	(9/15)	60%	(12/16)	75%	(12/20)	60%
Multiple lesions/vessel	(11/16)	69%	(11/19)	58%	(26/35)	74%	(26/30)	87%
Overall	(29/53)	55%	(29/53)	55%	(45/58)	78%	(45/58)	78%

The high negative predictive value in most studies suggests that the absence of disease can be diagnosed more confidently than the presence of a significant stenosis. According to some investigators, MSCT coronary angiography may therefore be more valuable as a tool to exclude significant lesions in patients with a relatively low pre-test likelihood for the presence of stenoses, and less for staging patients with a very high likelihood and expectedly advanced coronary artery degeneration (Figure 5.13).

PATIENT-BASED DIAGNOSTIC PERFORMANCE OF MSCT

The majority of studies report the diagnostic capabilities of CT based on coronary segment or coronary vessel analysis. However, to demonstrate clinical relevance assessment of the diagnostic performance of computed tomography on a per patient-based analysis may be preferred (Table 5.7). To date, only very few studies have reported the patient-based analysis approach[15,21].

CONSIDERATIONS AND LIMITATIONS

Despite significant technological progress and increasing experience with the evaluation of MSCT coronary angiography, a number of challenges remain (Table 5.8). Technical limitations in terms of spatial resolution, temporal resolution and contrast-to-noise have been discussed in previous chapters. As a consequence of these, some patient characteristics are unfavorable and are more likely to result in non-interpretable examinations. Image quality is poorer in patients with a fast or irregular heart rate. Coronary arteries with diffuse and calci-

Table 5.8 Unfavorable patient characteristics

Fast heart rate (>75 bpm)

Persistent irregular heart rhythm

Small coronary arteries

Diffuse and calcified coronary atheroscleroisis

Coronary stents

Metal objects: prosthetic valves, pacemaker wires, etc.

High body mass index

Respiratory impairment and related motion artifacts

Renal dysfunction and contrast medium allergy

fied atherosclerotic disease are more difficult to assess. A high body mass index results in more image noise and requires a higher roentgen dose. Contrast-enhanced MSCT is contraindicated in patients with impaired renal function or known allergy to iodine-containing contrast media. The considerable radiation dose remains a matter of concern and limits the application of this technique.

When coronary artery segments are regarded as evaluable, a number of misinterpretations continue to be made. Overestimation, and occasionally underestimation, of lesion severity can be caused by motion artifacts or be related to the lack of objective quantification tools, lack of a representative reference diameter, misuse of the window level and width settings (Figure 5.14), etc. Other reasons for stenosis overestimation include cardiac arrhythmia, which results in discontinuity of vessels in the longitudinal direction, giving the impression of an obstruction with three-dimensional post-processing applications. Highly attenuating materials, such as stents or plaques, cause blooming artifacts that create

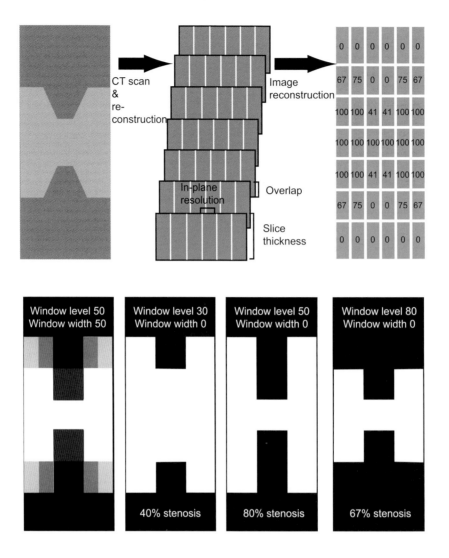

Figure 5.14 Stenosis severity depending on the window level/width settings. Imaging of small stenosed vessels with a limited spatial resolution is dependent on the window level and width settings. The vessel is scanned with a slice width of approximately one-half of the vessel width, for instance a 2.5-mm vessel with a 4×1-mm detector collimation (1.25-mm effective slice thickness). Reconstruction of overlapping slices results in density measurement that depends on the amount of contrast-enhanced lumen (100) and non-enhanced vessel wall (0). The stenosis severity varies with the varying window level and width settings

or exaggerate the apparent severity of stenosis (Figure 5.15). When the coronary arteries show severe and diffuse calcified atherosclerosis, MSCT angiography is not suitable[23]. It has been proposed that a non-enhanced calcium quantification scan should be performed first to exclude patients with an unfavorably high coronary calcium load, prior to contrast-enhanced CT angiography. In a number of overestimations by semiquantitatively assessed MSCT angiograms, lumenal narrowing is actually present but classified as less than significant with

computer-aided analysis of the conventional angiograms. In the study by Nieman *et al.* in seven out of 20 overestimated lesions by MSCT a subsignificant (40–49%) diameter reduction was present according to quantitative coronary angiography[21].

In our opinion, motion artifacts are currently the most important limitation of MSCT coronary angiography. They result in non-assessable investigations, and thereby reduce the clinical applicability of the technique. Two studies evaluated the diagnostic accuracy of

MSCT in relation to the heart rate of the patient. Giesler *et al.* divided 100 patients into four groups and showed that in patients with a heart rate below 60 bpm motion artifacts occurred in only 8% of the coronary arteries, compared to 18% at a heart rate between 61 and 70 bpm, 41% at between 71 and 80 bpm, and 22% of more than 80 bpm. The respective percentages of non-assessable vessels were 22%, 23%, 50% and 24%, which resulted in a decreasing overall sensitivity to detect > 70% coronary diameter narrowing in 67%, 55%, 35% and 22%, for the respective heart-rate groups[17]. In a study by Nieman *et al.* 78 patients were divided equally into three groups according to the average heart rate during MSCT coronary angiography[18]. In

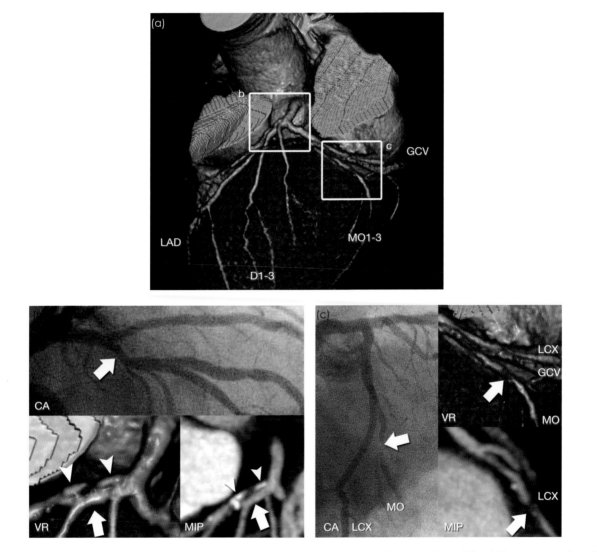

Figure 5.15 (a) Volume-rendered image (left lateral view) providing an anatomical overview of the left coronary artery. The boxes indicate the location of more-detailed images shown in Figure 5.15b and 5.15c. (b) Detailed image of the proximal left anterior descending coronary artery. Severe calcifications (arrowheads) cause blooming artifacts on CT and result in overestimation of the degree of stenosis. The invasive angiography image (CA) shows only a non-significant coronary lesion (arrow), whereas the volume-rendered (VR) and maximum-intensity projection (MIP) CT images suggest a (false positive) significant lesion (arrows). (c) Detailed image of the marginal obtuse (MO) branch. This lesion predominantly consists of non-calcified plaque tissue, and the CT images do not suffer from blooming artifacts. The invasive angiography image (CA) shows a significant lesion, which is also represented on the volume-rendered (VR) and maximum intensity projection (MIP) CT images. Note: the great cardiac vein (GCV) obscures the visualization of the proximal part of the MO on the volume-rendered image. LCX, left circumflex coronary artery; D1–3, first, second and third diagonal branch; GCV, great cardiac vein; LAD, left anterior descending coronary artery; MO1–3, first, second and third marginal branch

the low-heart rate group (56 ± 4 bpm), intermediate-heart rate group (67 ± 3 bpm), and high-heart rate group (82 ± 9 bpm), the number of assessable segments were 78%, 73% and 54%, resulting in an overall sensitivity to detect > 50% lumenal stenosis of 82%, 61% and 32%, respectively. The accuracy of MSCT to classify patients as having no, single or multivessel disease, without exclusion of non-assessable segments, was 73%, 54% and 42%, for each respective group (Figure 5.16)[18]. Based on experiences like these, many centers now routinely use anti-chronotropical medication, such as beta-blockers, particularly in patients with higher heart rates, to reduce the occurrence of motion artifacts, and improve the diagnostic accuracy of MSCT coronary angiography.

CLINICAL IMPLEMENTATION

A number of potential applications of MSCT coronary angiography have been listed in Table 5.9. For the detection or imaging of coronary stenosis MSCT is not as harmless and inexpensive as exercise electrocardiography, neither is it as accurate and informative as conventional coronary angiography. It may, however, fill a diagnostic niche between the relatively low diagnostic accuracy and ambiguity of exercise tests and the invasiveness and high cost of catheter-based techniques (Figure 5.17). In patients with a modest heart rate MSCT could provide a useful and reliable alternative to diagnostic catheter-based angiography for the initial detection and localization of coronary stenoses. Additionally, because of its non-invasive nature, MSCT coronary angiography can be introduced into the diagnostic work-up of patients with anginal complaints at an earlier stage, when catheter-based angiography is not yet indicated. Potential applications are the exclusion of coronary obstruction in cases of atypical or refractory chest pain and when a coronary origin of the symptoms is doubted or when non-invasive testing is (Figure 5.15) inconclusive. Also, in patients who need major (non-cardiac) surgery coronary artery disease can be excluded by CT angiography. MSCT may also be valuable when repeated angiographic follow-up is indicated, or after percutaneous coronary intervention or coronary artery bypass surgery (Table 5.9).

MSCT angiography can serve not only as a non-invasive alternative to conventional coronary angiography, it

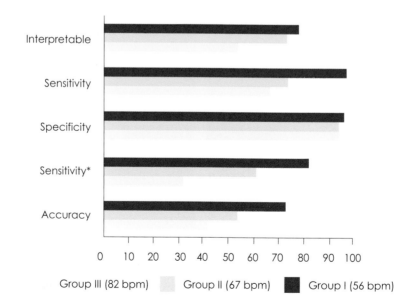

Figure 5.16 Heart rate dependent diagnostic performance of MSCT coronary angiography. Graph showing the image interpretability, the sensitivity and specificity to detect >50% stenosis in interpretable >2.0-mm coronary segments, the overall sensitivity including lesions in non-interpretable coronary segments, and accuracy to classify patients as having no significant lesions, single-vessel disease or multi-vessel disease, in patients with a low (56 bpm), intermediate (67 bpm) or high heart rate (82 bpm)

Table 5.9 Potential applications of CT coronary angiography

Early detection of stenosis

Non-symptomatic high-risk patients

Exclusion of stenosis
high-risk patients
prior to major (non-cardiac) surgery

Detection and/or exclusion of stenoses
atypical (unstable) chest pain
refractory chest pain with doubtful coronary origin
non-conclusive stress tests

Substitution of conventional coronary angiography
prior to percutaneous coronary intervention
high-risk patients: aortic disease

Adjuvant to coronary angiography
plaque characterization
complicated coronary intubation
total coronary occlusion

Follow-up
percutaneous coronary intervention
bypass surgery

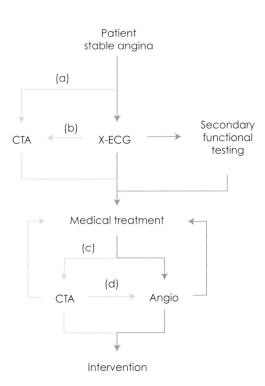

Figure 5.17 Potential application of CT angiography (CTA). (a) As an alternative to exercise stress testing (X-EGG). (b) Following a positive exercise stress test. (c) Patients refractory to medical treatment, who are scheduled for coronary angiography where CT coronary angiography may be an alternative to angiography. (d) CT coronary angiography followed by angiography

may also provide additional and possibly valuable information with respect to the coronary artery wall[25,26]. Another advantage of MSCT angiography is the possibility of presenting results in a three-dimensional fashion, which can be useful to show an anomaly[27], or to relate a coronary lesion to dysfunctioning or otherwise abnormal myocardial tissue[28].

CONCLUSION

CT coronary angiography is considered to be a significant breakthrough diagnostic modality to assess non-invasively the coronary lumen. It is expected that further technical improvements will soon be implemented to make this technique a reliable clinical diagnostic tool in a broad spectrum of patients. Problems remaining to be solved are reduction of cardiac motion artifacts associated with fast heart rates, the radiation exposure should be reduced and ways should be found to handle obscuring calcium image artifacts and, eventually, it should also be possible for patients with an irregular heart rhythm to be imaged. Many single and multicenter studies need to be performed in a wide spectrum of patients with different prevalences of coronary artery disease to demonstrate convincingly the safety and reliability of non-invasive CT coronary angiography in clinical practice.

REFERENCES

1. Moshage WE, Achenbach S, Seese B, et al. Coronary artery stenoses: three-dimensional imaging with electrocardiographically triggered, contrast agent-enhanced, electron-beam CT. Radiology 1995; 196: 707–14

2. Achenbach S, Moshage W, Ropers D, et al. Value of electron-beam computed tomography for the noninvasive detection of high-grade coronary-artery stenoses and occlusions. N Engl J Med 1998; 339: 1964–71

3. Rensing BJ, Bongaerts A, van Geuns RJ, et al. Intravenous coronary angiography by electron beam computed tomography: a clinical evaluation. Circulation 1998; 98: 2509–12

4. Reddy G, Chernoff DM, Adams JR, et al. Coronary artery stenoses: assessment with contrast-enhanced electron-beam CT and axial reconstructions. Radiology 1998; 208: 167–72

5. Schmermund A, Rensing BJ, Sheedy PF, et al. Intravenous electron-beam computed tomographic coronary angiography for segmental analysis of coronary artery stenoses. J Am Coll Cardiol 1998; 31: 1547–54

6. Nakanishi T, Ito K, Imazu M, et al. Evaluation of coronary artery stenoses using electron-beam CT and multiplanar reformation. J Comput Assist Tomogr 1997; 21: 121–7

7. Budoff MJ, Oudiz RJ, Zalace CP, et al. Intravenous three-dimensional coronary angiography using contrast-enhanced electron beam computed tomography. Am J Cardiol 1999; 83: 840–5

8. Moshage W, Ropers D, Daniel WG, Achenbach S. [Noninvasive imaging of coronary arteries with electron beam tomography (EBCT).] Z Kardiol 2000; 89 (Suppl 1): 15–20

9. Achenbach S, Ropers D, Regenfus M, et al. Contrast enhanced electron beam computed tomography to analyse the coronary arteries in patients after acute myocardial infarction. Heart 2000; 84: 489–93

10. Lu B, Zhuang N, Mao SS, et al. Image quality of three-dimensional electron beam coronary angiography. J Comput Assist Tomogr 2002; 26: 202–9

11. Nieman K, Oudkerk M, Rensing BJ, et al. Coronary angiography with multi-slice computed tomography. Lancet 2001; 357: 599–603

12. Achenbach S, Giesler T, Ropers D, et al. Detection of coronary artery stenoses by contrast-enhanced, retrospectively electrocardiographically-gated, multislice spiral computed tomography. Circulation 2001; 103: 2535–8

13. Knez A, Becker CR, Leber A, et al. Usefulness of multislice spiral computed tomography angiography for determination of coronary artery stenoses. Am J Cardiol 2001; 88: 1191–4

14. Vogl TJ, Abolmaali ND, Diebold T, et al. Techniques for the detection of coronary atherosclerosis: multidetector row CT coronary angiography. Radiology 2002; 223: 212–20

15. Nieman K, Rensing BJ, van Geuns RJM, et al. Usefulness of multislice computed tomography for detecting obstructive coronary artery disease. Am J Cardiol 2002; 89: 913–18

16. Kopp AF, Schröder S, Küttner A, et al. Non-invasive coronary angiography with high resolution multidetector-row computed tomography: results in 102 patients. Eur Heart J 2002; 23: 1714–25

17. Giesler T, Baum U, Ropers D, et al. Noninvasive visualization of coronary arteries using contrast-enhanced multidetector CT: influence of heart rate on image quality and stenosis detection. Am J Roentgenol 2002; 179: 911–16

18. Nieman K, Rensing BJ, van Geuns RJ, et al. Non-invasive coronary angiography with multislice spiral computed tomography: impact of heart rate. Heart 2002; 88: 470–4

19. Kuettner A, Kopp AF, Schroeder S, et al. Diagnostic accuracy of multidetector computed tomography coronary angiography in patients with angiographically proven coronary artery disease. J Am Coll Cardiol 2004; 43: 831–9

20. Maruyama T, Yoshizumi T, Tamura R, et al. Comparison of visibility and diagnostic capability of noninvasive coronary angiography by eight-slice multidetector-row computed tomography versus conventional coronary angiography. Am J Cardiol 2004; 93: 537–42

21. Nieman K, Cademartiri F, Lemos PA, et al. Reliable noninvasive coronary angiography with fast submillimeter multislice spiral computed tomography. Circulation 2002; 106: 2051–4

22. Ropers D, Baum U, Pohle K, et al. Detection of coronary artery stenoses with thin-slice multi-detector row spiral computed tomography and multiplanar reconstruction. Circulation 2003; 107: 664–6

23. Kuettner A, Trabold T, Schroeder S, et al. Non-invasive detection of coronary lesions using 16-slice MDCT technology: initial clinical results. J Am Coll Cardiol 2004; in press

24. Mollet NR, Cademartiri F, Nieman K, et al. Multislice spiral CT coronary angiography in patients with stable angina pectoris. J Am Coll Cardiol 2004; 43: 2265–70

25. Schroeder S, Kopp AF, Baumbach A, et al. Noninvasive detection and evaluation of atherosclerotic coronary plaques with multislice computed tomography. J Am Coll Cardiol 2001; 37: 1430–5

26. Achenbach S, Moselewski F, Ropers D, et al. Detection of calcified and noncalcified coronary atherosclerotic plaque by contrast-enhanced, submillimeter multidetector spiral computed tomography: a segment-based comparison with intravascular ultrasound. Circulation 2004; 109: 14–17

27. Ropers D, Gehling G, Pohle K, et al. Anomalous course of the left main or left anterior descending coronary artery originating from the right sinus of Valsalva. Identification of four common variations by electron beam tomography. Circulation 2002; 105: e42–3

28. Dirksen MS, Bax JJ, de Roos A, et al. Usefulness of dynamic multislice computed tomography and left ventricular function in unstable angina pectoris and comparison with echocardiography. Am J Cardiol 2002; 90: 1157–60

CHAPTER 6

Coronary plaque imaging

Direct non-invasive imaging of coronary calcific and non-calcific atherosclerotic plaques may significantly improve risk stratification of adverse coronary events and may prove useful in the better understanding of the development and progression of coronary atherosclerosis.

COMPOSITION OF CORONARY PLAQUES ASSESSED BY MSCT

The recently introduced 16-slice spiral CT scanner is able to identify advanced coronary plaques. These plaques can be either non-obstructive due to arterial wall compensatory remodeling or may impact on the coronary lumen (Figure 6.1). The 16-slice MSCT scanner permits assessment of the extent, severity and localization of coronary plaques[1–10]. Furthermore, the 16-slice MSCT scanner can distinguish between the various components of advanced plaques which have different X-ray density values. Lipid and fibrous tissue are low-density structures and calcium is a high-density structure, whereas a very low-density obstruction in the setting of an acute coronary syndrome may represent a thrombotic occlusion (Figures 6.2–6.5). Moreover, it has been shown that MSCT on the basis of differences in density values between non-calcific plaques could distinguish between lipid and fibrous plaques, which may have an impact on the identification of high-risk coronary plaques.

In a comparative study of the histology and *in vivo* MSCT imaging of large carotid plaques in patients who underwent carotid endarterectomy, CT scanning was able to distinguish between lipid tissue that had a mean attenuation value of 39 ± 12 HU and fibrous tissue with a mean value of 90 ± 24 HU[10]. Schroeder *et al.* were the

first to demonstrate that distinction between lipid and fibrous plaques was also possible in smaller coronary plaques[2]. These results were confirmed by the study of Leber *et al.* who, in a elegant study, demonstrated that the density measurements between lipid and fibrous plaques were different[11] (Table 6.1). Both studies correlated the coronary lesion echogenicity of intravascular ultrasound (IVUS) and computed tomography density measurement, thereby taking IVUS as the reference standard to distinguish between lipid and fibrous tissue. It is of note that IVUS does not equate with histology; however, it is the best possible assumption in the setting of *in vivo* coronary plaque imaging.

DETECTION OF CORONARY PLAQUES BY MSCT

The diagnostic value of MSCT to detect coronary plaques has been reported for non-calcific and calcific plaques[7,11]. The sensitivity was dependent on the plaque composition with lower sensitivity for non-calcified plaques and very high sensitivity for calcified plaques (Table 6.2). The specificity ranged from 88% to 92%. Plaques that were not detected were smaller and located in smaller vessels (Table 6.3).

Nikolaou *et al.* reported the prevalence of coronary calcific and non-calcific plaques in 179 patients. Coronary calcific lesions were detected in 73% of the patients and non-calcific plaques were seen in 30%[3].

Leber *et al.* reported the distribution of calcific, mixed and non-calcific plaques in 19 patients with stable angina and in 21 patients who survived an acute myocardial infarction (Table 6.4)[5]. The acute myocardial infarction patients had fewer calcific and more non-calcific lesions than the stable angina patients.

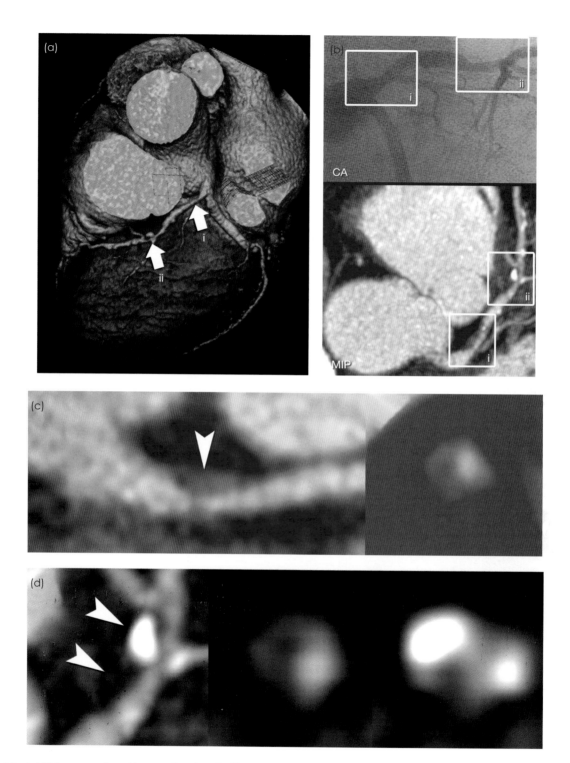

Figure 6.1 (a) Volume-rendered image showing significant obstructive lesions in the proximal and mid-part of the left anterior descending coronary artery (arrows i and ii). (b) Invasive diagnostic angiogram (CA) and corresponding maximum-intensity projection MSCT image (MIP). The lesions are highlighted in boxes (i) and (ii). MSCT coronary angiography provides not only information regarding the coronary lumen but also about coronary plaques: non-calcific plaque (i) and mixed (calcific/non-calcific) plaque (ii). (c) Multiplanar reconstructed image (left panel) of the proximal coronary lesion showing a non-calcified plaque. The arrowhead indicates the location of the cross-sectional image of the plaque (right panel), again showing the contrast-enhanced lumen and adjacent non-calcified plaque tissue. (d) Multiplanar reconstructed image (left panel) of the distal coronary lesion showing a mixed plaque. The arrowheads indicate cross-sectional images of the plaque at the level of the non-calcified plaque tissue (middle panel) and the calcified plaque tissue (right panel)

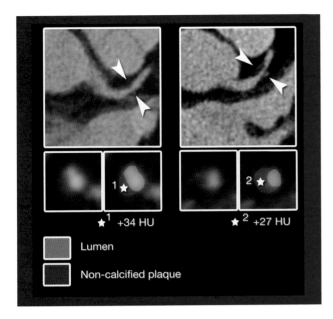

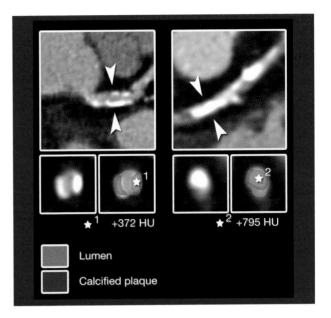

Figure 6.2 Non-significant (left panels) and significant obstructive (right panels) non-calcified plaques. The arrowheads indicate the location of cross-sectional images of the plaques (lower panels). The HU values measured within the plaques are in the range of lipid plaque tissue

Figure 6.3 Non-significant (left panels) and significant obstructive (right panels) mixed plaques. The arrowheads indicate the location of cross-sectional images of the plaques (lower panels), showing the presence of both non-calcified (a) and calcified (b) plaque tissue components

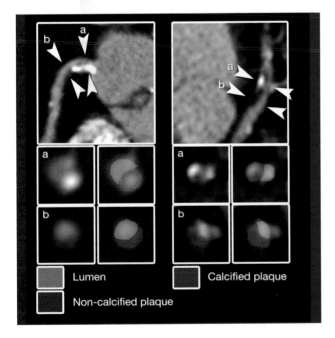

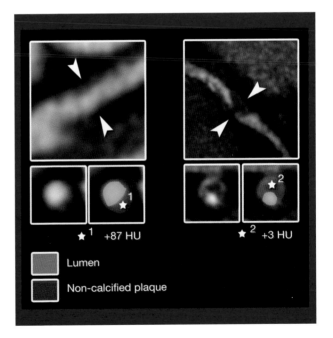

Figure 6.4 Non-significant (left panels) and significant obstructive (right panels) calcified plaques. The arrowheads indicate the location of cross-sectional images of the plaques (lower panels). The HU values measured within the plaques are in the range of calcified plaque tissue

Figure 6.5 Non-significant (left panels) and significant obstructive (right panels) non-calcified plaques. The arrowheads indicate the location of cross-sectional images of the plaques (lower panels). The HU values measured within the non-significant lesion are in the range of fibrous plaque tissue. However, the HU values measured within the significant lesion in this patient with unstable angina suggest the presence of a thrombotic plaque

Table 6.1 Plaque composition with contrast-enhanced CT coronary plaque imaging

	MSCT study	
IVUS	Schroeder et al.[2] (HU ± SD) (n = 17)	Leber et al.[11] (HU ± SD) (n = 37)
Hypoechoic	14 ± 26	49 ± 22
Hyperechoic	91 ± 21	91 ± 22
Calcified	419 ± 194	391 ± 156

IVUS, intravascular ultrasound

Table 6.2 Diagnostic value of MSCT to detect coronary plaques

IVUS plaque	Achenbach et al.[7] (n = 22) sensitivity		IVUS	Leber et al.[11] (n = 37) sensitivity	
Mixed	78%	(35/45)	hypoechoic	78%	(62/80)
Non-calcific	53%	(8/15)	hyperechoic	78%	(87/112)
Calcified	92%	(33/36)	calcified	95%	(150/158)
Any plaque	82%	(41/50)	any plaque	86%	(299/350)
Exclusion plaque (specificity)	88%	(29/33)		92%	(484/525)

Table 6.3 MSCT: characteristics of detected and non-detected plaques

	Non-detected plaques	Detected plaques
Plaque thickness (mm)	0.9 ± 0.3	1.5 ± 0.3
External diameter (mm)	3.6 ± 1.1	4.5 ± 1.2
Plaque volume (mm^3)	47 ± 11	76 ± 10
Plaque area (mm^2)	8 ± 3	11 ± 4

Table 6.4 Prevalence of MSCT coronary plaque types[4]

	Stable angina (n = 19)	Acute myocardial infarction (n = 21)
Plaques/patient (n)	12 ± 6	10 ± 5
Calcific plaque (%)	79	56
Mixed plaque (%)	13	18
Non-calcific plaque (%)	7	24

Mollet *et al.* investigated 78 patients with MSCT to assess the MSCT-determined coronary plaque burden, which was defined as plaque extent, distribution, severity and type of plaque. The results and an example of a patient with a high MSCT coronary plaque burden are shown in Figures 6.6–6.9[9].

REMODELING OF CORONARY PLAQUE

Coronary artery wall expansive remodeling occurs in the earlier phases of the development of coronary atherosclerosis, and enlargement of the total vessel tends to preserve the normal size of the coronary lumen.

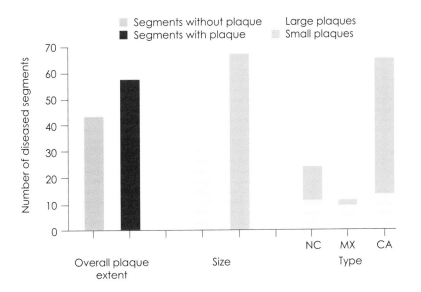

Figure 6.6 Results of plaque extent (number of diseased segments), size (large or small), type (non-calcified (NC), mixed (MX) and calcified (CA)), and number of plaques per patient assessed with MSCT coronary angiography in 78 patients with stable angina pectoris yielding a total of 855 segments. Overall, there were 6.2±2.9 plaques per patient

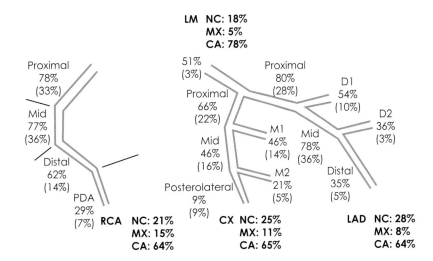

Figure 6.7 Distribution of any plaque and large plaques (in brackets) within the coronary segments. Plaque type is shown per vessel. Plaques are predominantly located in the proximal and mid-segments of the main coronary vessels. NC, non-calcified plaque; MX, mixed plaque; CA, calcified plaque; D1, first diagonal branch; D2, second diagonal branch; M1, first marginal branch; M2, second marginal branch; LM, left main coronary artery; LAD, left anterior descending coronary artery; CX, circumflex coronary artery; PDA, posterior descending artery

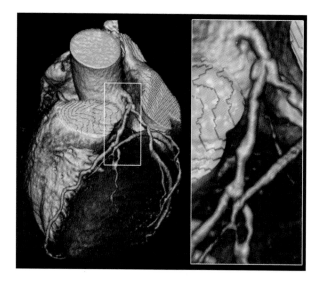

Figure 6.8 Volume-rendered image of a patient with a high plaque burden in the left anterior descending coronary artery assessed with MSCT coronary angiography. This image-processing technique only provides information regarding the coronary lumen and coronary calcifications, whereas non-calcified plaque tissue components are not visualized

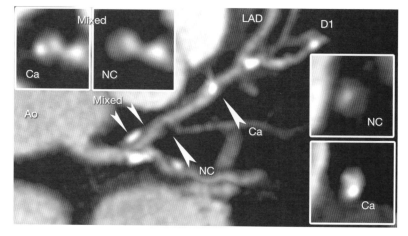

Figure 6.9 Maximum-intensity projection and cross-sectional multiplanar reconstructed (inserts) MSCT images of the left main and proximal part of the left anterior descending coronary artery (LAD) of the same patient. The LAD is severely diseased and different types of plaques are visualized including mixed, calcified (Ca) and non-calcified (NC) plaques. Ao, aorta; D1, first diagonal branch. Arrowheads denote site of cross-sectional images

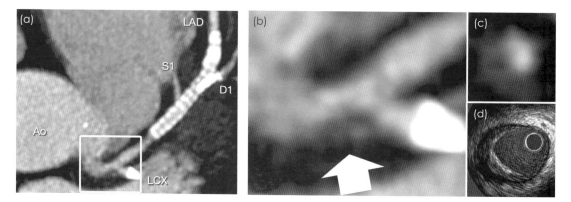

Figure 6.10 Maximum-intensity images of the left main and proximal part of the left anterior descending coronary artery (LAD) (a) and (b). The box highlights a non-calcified plaque at the level of the left main and the bifurcation, without encroachment of the coronary lumen, which is also shown in (c) (cross-sectional image of the plaque). These MSCT findings were confirmed with intracoronary ultrasound (d). The vessel shows positive (expansive) remodeling. Ao, aorta; D1, first diagonal branch; LCX, left circumflex coronary artery; S1, segment branch 1

Achenbach *et al.* demonstrated that MSCT can identify coronary plaques with positive (expansive) vessel wall remodeling and negative (shrinkage) remodeling (Figure 6.10)[8].

MSCT IDENTIFICATION OF VULNERABLE PLAQUES

It has been shown that plaque composition, morphology and expansive coronary wall remodeling may be more important predictors of plaque vulnerability and clinical behavior than the degree of coronary stenosis[12-18].

Non-invasive MSCT plaque imaging can play a role in the identification of a high-risk plaque. This can be illustrated in the case history of a patient who was admitted with transient acute chest pain and ECG changes (Figure 6.11). The MSCT coronary angiogram showed a non-significant mid-LAD lesion as did the diagnostic invasive coronary angiogram. Non-invasive MSCT clearly showed a non-calcific plaque with vessel

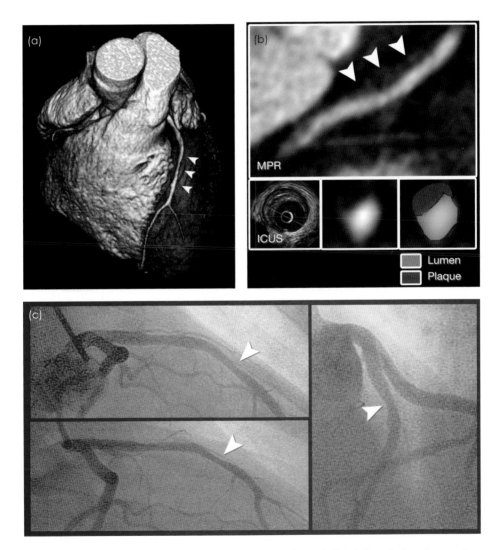

Figure 6.11 (a) Volume-rendered image showing only mild narrowing of the left anterior descending coronary artery (arrowheads), whereas the other coronary arteries were completely normal (not shown). (b) Multiplanar reconstructed image (MPR) of the proximal left anterior descending coronary artery. The arrowheads indicate the presence of a non-calcified plaque with positive vessel remodeling, which was confirmed with intracoronary ultrasound (ICUS). Cross-sectional MSCT images also show the presence of a non-calcified plaque without encroachment of the lumen (lower right panels). (c) Invasive coronary angiogram confirming the presence of a non-significant lesion in the proximal part of the left anterior descending coronary artery in different projections

remodeling, which was confirmed with intracoronary ultrasound.

LIMITATIONS OF MSCT PLAQUE IMAGING

The resolution of the current MSCT scanners fails to detect the very early stages of coronary atherosclerosis development. More advanced coronary plaques can be detected, but MSCT substantially underestimates the plaque volume as compared with intracoronary ultrasound[7]. The volume of calcific plaques may be overestimated owing to partial voluming, and there often appears to be a dark circumferential artifact around the calcium which obscures identification of the adjacent tissue and, thus, may underestimate the presence of mixed plaques, and does not allow plaques with deep or superficial layers of calcium to be distinguished as can be seen by intracoronary ultrasound.

CONCLUSION

Non-invasive CT assessment of the coronary plaque burden appears to be a useful addition to the diagnostic armamentarium in cardiological practice (Table 6.5). It will increase our understanding of the development and progression of coronary atherosclerosis, and it may carry additional prognostic information. In patients with moderate- to high-quality MSCT images (poor-quality images were excluded), comparative studies with IVUS demonstrated that calcified plaques can be detected with a high sensitivity (> 90%), but non-calcified plaque detection was less reliable with sensitivities ranging from 53% to 78%. The specificity ranged between 88% and 92%. Smaller non-calcific plaques were not reliably detected and the volume and area of plaques were significantly underestimated.

Non-invasive CT assessment of coronary plaques of the clinically relevant parts of the entire coronary tree (as opposed to intracoronary diagnostic tools) may be useful in the identification of a vulnerable plaque (Table 6.6). Non-invasive detection may further guide invasive diagnostic tools. Early non-invasive detection of coronary plaques may eventually improve management of both individuals with subclinically coronary artery disease and asymptomatic patients with known coronary artery disease.

Table 6.5 CT coronary plaque imaging

Non-contrast enhanced imaging (EBCT-MSCT): coronary calcium quantification
Predict presence of significant coronary obstruction
Risk stratification

Contrast-enhanced imaging (MSCT): coronary lumen and plaque imaging
Number of plaques (extent)
Plaque distribution (RCA, left main, LAD, LCX)
Plaque type
   calcific
   non-calcific
   mixed
   thrombotic in ACS
Lumen obstruction
   non-obstructive
   ≥ 50%
   total occlusion
Vessel wall remodeling
May have improved risk stratification?

EBCT, electron-beam CT; MSCT, multislice CT; RCA, right coronary artery; LAD, left anterior descending artery; LCX, left circumflex artery; ACS, acute coronary syndrome

Table 6.6 Vulnerable plaque features: non-invasive and invasive diagnosis

	MSCT	Invasive tools
Plaque components		
lipid	low density	angioscopy/IVUS
fibrous	moderate density	IVUS
calcific	high density	IVUS
Severe narrowing	+	coronary angiography
Remodeling	±	IVUS
Fibrous cap	–	OCT
Inflammation	–	thermography
Deformability	–	palpography

IVUS, intravascular ultrasound; OCT, optical coherence tomography

REFERENCES

1. Becker CR, Knez A, Ohnesorge B, et al. Imaging of noncalcified coronary plaques using helical CT with retrospective ECG gating. Am J Roentgenol 2000; 175: 423–4

2. Schroeder S, Kopp AF, Baumbach A, et al. Noninvasive detection and evaluation of atherosclerotic coronary plaques with multislice computed tomography. J Am Coll Cardiol 2001; 37: 1430–5

3. Nikolaou K, Sagmeister S, Knez A, et al. Multidetector-row computed tomography of the coronary arteries: predictive value and quantitative assessment of non-calcified vessel-wall changes. Eur Radiol 2003; 13: 2505–12

4. Leber AW, Knez A, White CW, et al. Composition of coronary atherosclerotic plaques in patients with acute myocardial infarction and stable angina pectoris determined by contrast-enhanced multislice computed tomography. Am J Cardiol 2003; 91: 714–18

5. Caussin C, Ohanessian A, Lancelin B, et al. Coronary plaque burden detected by multislice computed tomography after acute myocardial infarction with near-normal coronary arteries by angiography. Am J Cardiol 2003; 92: 849–52

6. Becker CR, Nikolaou K, Muders M, et al. Ex vivo coronary atherosclerotic plaque characterization with multidetector-row CT. Eur Radiol 2003; 13: 2094–8

7. Achenbach S, Moselewski F, Ropers D, et al. Detection of calcified and noncalcified coronary atherosclerotic plaque by contrast-enhanced, submillimeter multidetector spiral computed tomography: a segment-based comparison with intravascular ultrasound. Circulation 2004; 109: 14–17

8. Achenbach S, Ropers D, Hoffmann U, et al. Assessment of coronary remodeling in stenotic and nonstenotic coronary atherosclerotic lesions by multidetector spiral computed tomography. J Am Coll Cardiol 2004; 43: 842–7

9. Mollet NRA, et al. 2004; submitted

10. Estes JM, Quist WC, Lo Gerfo FW, Costello P. Noninvasive characterization of plaque morphology using helical computed tomography. J Cardiovasc Surg (Torino) 1998; 39: 527–34

11. Leber AW, Knez A, Becker A, et al. Accuracy of multidetector spiral computed tomography in identifying and differentiating the composition of coronary atherosclerotic plaques; a comparative study with intracoronary ultrasound. J Am Coll Cardiol 2004; 43: 1241–7

12. Varnava AM, Mills PG, Davies MJ. Relationship between coronary artery remodeling and plaque vulnerability. Circulation 2002; 105: 939–43

13. Pasterkamp G, Schoneveld AH, van der Wal AC, et al. Relation of arterial geometry to luminal narrowing and histologic markers for plaque vulnerability: the remodeling paradox. J Am Coll Cardiol 1998; 32: 655–62

14. Takano M, Mizuno K, Okamatsu K, et al. Mechanical and structural characteristics of vulnerable plaques: analysis by coronary angioscopy and intravascular ultrasound. J Am Coll Cardiol 2001; 38: 99–104

15. Nakamura M, Nishikawa H, Mukai S, et al. Impact of coronary artery remodeling on clinical presentation of coronary artery disease: an intravascular ultrasound study. J Am Coll Cardiol 2001; 37: 63–9

16. Schoenhagen P, Ziada KM, Kapadia SR, et al. Extent and direction of arterial remodeling in stable versus unstable coronary syndromes: an intravascular ultrasound study. Circulation 2000; 101: 598–603

17. Schoenhagen P, Tuzcu EM, Stillman AE, et al. Noninvasive assessment of plaque morphology and remodeling in mildly stenotic coronary segments: comparison of 16-slice computed tomography and intravascular ultrasound. Coron Artery Dis 2003; 14: 459–62

18. Gyongyosi M, Yang P, Hassan A, et al. Intravascular ultrasound predictors of major adverse cardiac events in patients with unstable angina. Clin Cardiol 2000; 23: 507–15

CHAPTER 7

Coronary calcification

Imaging of coronary arteries has been a major focus of clinicians interested in cardiovascular disease for a long time. The search for, in particular, non-invasive methods has led to the development of electron-beam computed tomography (EBCT), a non-invasive imaging modality, which is able to detect coronary calcification. The recently introduced multislice CT (MSCT) scanners, which have an improved resolution, are able to detect both calcific and non-calcific plaques[1-8]. No long-term risk stratification studies are available using MSCT; however, it is expected that direct non-invasive imaging of coronary calcific and non-calcific atherosclerotic plaques may potentially improve risk stratification for asymptomatic individuals or in patients with known coronary artery disease.

CORONARY CALCIFICATION

The need to detect coronary atherosclerosis early in its course has been well recognized by cardiologists for decades. Better non-invasive methods, in particular, are needed to identify individuals whose first symptom of coronary artery disease is sudden death or myocardial infarction. The presence and amount of coronary artery calcium have been suggested as a means to assess patients at risk of adverse coronary events. Comparative anatomic and intravascular studies have shown that the presence of coronary calcium is always indicative of the presence of coronary atherosclerosis[1-9].

For many years, EBCT has been used for the detection and quantification of coronary calcium. Coronary calcium deposits have a high X-ray density which is approximately 2–10-fold higher than the low-density adjacent non-calcific tissue and surrounding fat tissue. Agatston *et al.* developed a calcium scoring algorithm

for EBCT images that is now widely used in research and clinical practice (Figure 7.1)[10]. The calcium score is derived from the product of the area of calcification (mm^2) and a factor determined by the maximal X-ray density within that area. The area of calcification should be at least $1 mm^2$ and the X-ray density should exceed the threshold of 130 HU. The calcium score can be calculated per coronary segment, per coronary vessel (right coronary artery, left anterior descending, left circumflex artery) or for the entire coronary tree.

The prevalence and extent of coronary calcium varies widely from no calcium to a large amount of calcium (Figures 7.2–7.4) and increases with age in both men and women. In women there appears to be a lag time of 10 years in calcium deposition compared to men, whereas men in general have higher calcium scores than women (Table 7.1)[11]. Men and women with diabetes mellitus or markers of insulin resistance have an increased extent of coronary calcification (Table 7.2)[12].

CORONARY CALCIUM AS A PROGNOSTIC INDICATOR

The prognostic value of coronary calcium in asymptomatic subjects has been investigated in several large-scale studies (Table 7.3)[13-18]. These studies indicated that calcium scoring can be used as a risk factor and, in particular, a high calcium score, adjusted for age and gender, is associated with a relatively high risk of adverse coronary events (Figures 7.5 and 7.6). It remains difficult to draw definite conclusions from these studies because there may have been important selection bias. In some studies subjects were self-referrals, or responders to advertisement. Also, in other studies, coronary risk factors were not actually measured but

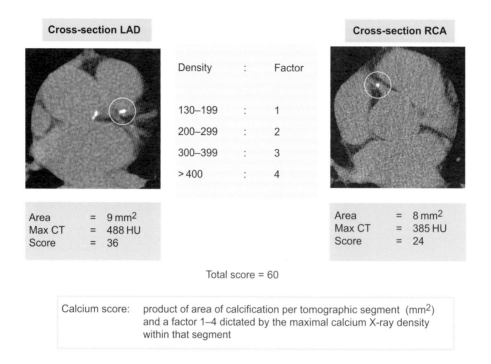

Cross-section LAD

Density	:	Factor
130–199	:	1
200–299	:	2
300–399	:	3
> 400	:	4

Cross-section RCA

Area	=	9 mm^2
Max CT	=	488 HU
Score	=	36

Area	=	8 mm^2
Max CT	=	385 HU
Score	=	24

Total score = 60

Calcium score: product of area of calcification per tomographic segment (mm^2) and a factor 1–4 dictated by the maximal calcium X-ray density within that segment

Figure 7.1 Coronary calcium scoring – Agatston score. LAD, left anterior descending artery; RCA, right coronary artery

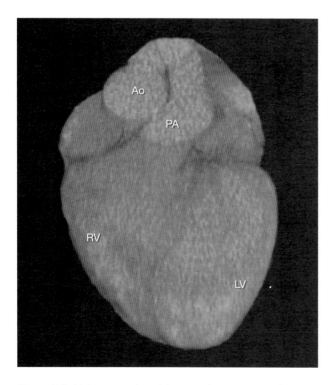

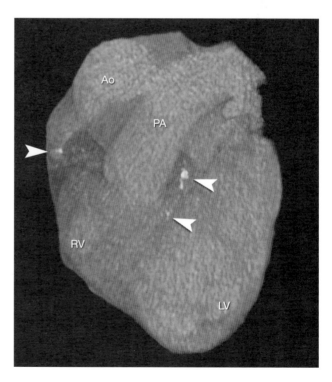

Figure 7.2 Volume-rendered image shows no calcium. LV, left ventricle; RV, right ventricle; Ao, aorta; PA, pulmonary artery

Figure 7.3 Volume-rendered image shows a small amount of calcium in left anterior descending and right coronary artery (arrows). LV, left ventricle; RV, right ventricle; Ao, aorta; PA, pulmonary artery

were estimated based on patient self-report. Furthermore, the follow-up period is relatively short, the number of hard events (death and myocardial infarction) is low and the number of patients without follow-up data is sometimes substantial, while some earlier reports included revascularizations among the coronary events counted to increase study power.

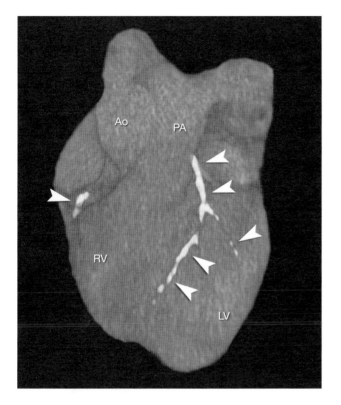

Figure 7.4 Volume-rendered image shows severely calcific left anterior descending and proximal right coronary artery (arrows). LV, left ventricle; RV, right ventricle; Ao, aorta; PA, pulmonary artery

HOW TO USE THE CALCIUM SCORE

CT calcium quantification can be used for the assessment of long-term risk and primary prevention of future adverse coronary events. However, calcium scoring should not be performed as a 'stand-alone' test but should be integrated into risk assessment with well-recognized risk factors (Table 7.4). Asymptomatic individuals can be categorized into three levels of risk[19–25]. Individuals considered to be at high risk are defined as having a risk of 20% or more of a coronary event within 10 years. This risk is similar to the level of risk in patients with known coronary artery disease, and according to the guidelines from the National Cholesterol Education Program (NCEP) this risk level is a target for intensive cholesterol reduction[19]. It is estimated that approximately 25% of adults in western countries fall into this category[22,23]. Intermediate risk is defined as the risk of a coronary event of 10–20% within 10 years and about 40% of the adults over 20 years of age fall into this category. Low risk is defined as a risk of a coronary event within 10 years of less than 10%. About 35% of adults over 20 years of age have low risk[22,23].

In the assessment of asymptomatic individuals coronary calcium scoring, in order to be useful, must be able to improve the prediction of the risk of coronary events, as established with known risk factors. It may be assumed that, because the calcium scoring test is not 100% sensitive and specific for the prediction of future adverse coronary events, a positive test will not be able to increase the risk of the pre-scan low-risk individuals to a high-risk category requiring preventive measures[19,24]. Furthermore, a negative calcium scan in a pre-

Table 7.1 EBCT calcium score centiles for 25 251 men and 9995 women within age strata. Reproduced from Hoff et al.[11], with permission

Calcium scores	Age (years)								
	<40	40–44	45–49	50–54	55–59	60–64	65–69	70–74	>74
Men (n)	3504	4238	4940	4825	3472	2288	1209	540	235
25th centile	0	0	0	1	4	13	32	64	166
50th centile	1	1	3	15	48	113	180	310	473
75th centile	3	9	36	103	215	410	566	892	1071
90th centile	14	59	154	332	554	994	1299	1774	1982
Women (n)	641	1024	1634	2184	1835	1334	731	438	174
25th centile	0	0	0	0	0	0	1	3	9
50th centile	0	0	0	0	1	3	24	52	75
75th centile	1	1	2	5	23	57	145	210	241
90th centile	3	4	22	55	121	193	410	631	709

Table 7.2 Median coronary artery calcium (CAC) scores of men and women with and without diabetes[12]

Age group (years)	Diabetes		No diabetes		p value
	n	Median CAC score	n	Median CAC score	
Men					
< 40	46	4	3005	1	< 0.001
40–44	63	13	3653	1	< 0.001
45–49	100	9.5	4322	3	0.001
50–54	144	42	4142	14	< 0.001
55–59	160	111	2192	43	< 0.001
60–64	117	192	1860	105	< 0.001
65–69	72	378	955	152	< 0.001
≥70	45	343	592	301	0.77
Total	747	63	20721	6	< 0.001
Women					
< 40	21	1	514	0	< 0.001
40–44	32	0	846	0	0.14
45–49	32	1	1398	0	0.01
50–54	74	8.5	1826	0	< 0.001
55–59	52	7.5	1522	1	< 0.001
60–64	47	21	1105	2	0.003
65–69	34	104	712	5	0.006
≥70	36	114	465	52	0.54
Total	328	5	8388	1	< 0.001

Mann-Whitney *U* test was used to compare CAC scores between diabetic and non-diabetic subjects within each 5-year age group. The analyses were performed separately for men and women

Table 7.3 Coronary calcium to predict adverse cardiac events

Study	n	Mean age (years)	Follow-up (years)	Gender (% male)	Events	Calcium score cut-off (n)	Risk ratio*
Wong et al.[13]	926	54	3.3	79	28	>81–270 >271	4.5* 8.8*
Arad et al.[17]	1172	53	3.7	71	18	≥160	22.2
Detrano et al.[14]	1196	66	3.4	89	44	> 44	2.3*
Raggi et al.[16]	676	52	2.7	51	30	>100	> 4.1%**
Kondos et al.[18]	5635	51	3.1	74	222	≥0	men 10.5 women 2.6

*Compared to patients with 0 score; **annualized event rate

scan high-risk population will not reduce this risk to a level at which preventive interventions could be withheld[19,24]. However, a calcium scan may be useful in the group of individuals with intermediate risk. Here, a positive or negative calcium scan may reclassify individuals to a higher- or lower-risk group, respectively, and thus provide further support for either instituting or withholding long-term preventive measures (Figure 7.7)[26].

Greenland and Gaziano in a landmark article presented a practical approach taking into account a pretest risk assessment and how the outcome of a calcium scan can influence clinical decision-making[27]. A pretest risk assessment can be derived from the risk assessment of the Framingham Heart Study or the European guidelines on cardiovascular disease prevention in clinical practice[19,28]. Greenland and Gaziano provided a

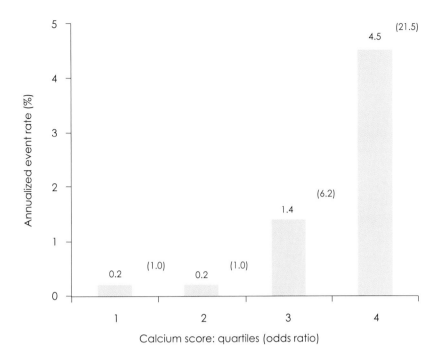

Figure 7.5 Quartiles of calcium score and annualized adverse coronary event rate. From reference 16, with permission

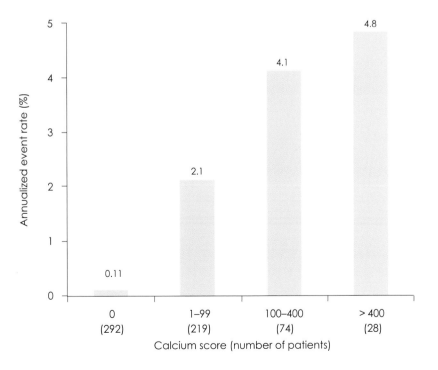

Figure 7.6 Calcium score and annualized adverse coronary event rate. From reference 16, with permission

straightforward, simple way to assess risk by counting risk factors. Individuals with zero or one risk factor are considered to be at low risk < 10% within 10 years, and individuals with three or more risk factors or diabetics are considered at high risk > 20% within 10 years[27]. It has been shown that a calcium score of more than 80 has a sensitivity of 85% and a specificity of 75% to predict the occurrence of clinical coronary events including death, non-fatal myocardial infarction and clinically indicated revascularization[17]. According to the calculations of Greenland and Gaziano a calcium score of less than 80 significantly reduced the risk of a coronary event within 10 years in the intermediate-risk group to less than 5% and, thus, to no need for preventive risk measures, whereas a calcium score of more than 80 significantly increased the risk in the intermediate-risk group to > 20% and, thus, to a category of individuals where preventive measures are warranted (Table 7.5). A

recent study demonstrated that a high calcium score was associated with independent additional risk in an intermediate-risk group as determined by the Framingham risk score[29]. This lends further support to the theory that a high calcium score can modify predicted risk, which is useful in an intermediate-risk group.

This approach is in accord with the statement of the Writing Group which suggested that in individuals at intermediate risk a calcium score may be useful to adjust classification of the individual to a lower-risk category if there is no calcium, or to a higher-risk category if calcium is present[26].

In conclusion, the presence of coronary calcium is a predictor of adverse coronary events. Calcification is neither a marker for plaque vulnerability nor for plaque stability. However, the greater is the overall calcium burden, which correlates with a greater overall coronary plaque burden, the greater is the likelihood of an adverse coronary event. The absence of calcium does not exclude the presence of coronary atherosclerosis but is associated with a low likelihood of advanced coronary atherosclerosis and a very low likelihood of an adverse coronary event. However, the data about the independent prognostic value of calcium, in addition to the traditional risk factors, yielded conflicting evidence[7]. The American College of Cardiology (ACC)/American Heart Association (AHA) consensus conference does not rec-

Table 7.4 Coronary risk factors in asymptomatic individuals

Non-adjustable risk factors	Adjustable risk factors
Sex	blood lipids
Age	smoking
Family history	diabetes
	blood pressure
	weight

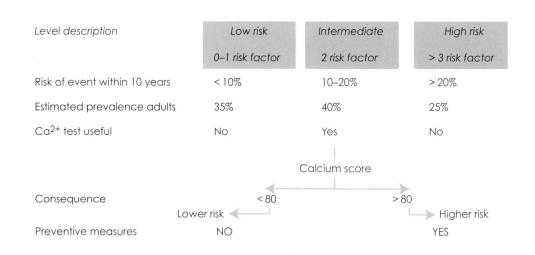

Level description	Low risk 0–1 risk factor	Intermediate 2 risk factor	High risk > 3 risk factor
Risk of event within 10 years	< 10%	10–20%	> 20%
Estimated prevalence adults	35%	40%	25%
Ca^{2+} test useful	No	Yes	No
		Calcium score	
Consequence	< 80		> 80
	Lower risk		Higher risk
Preventive measures	NO		YES

Figure 7.7 Approach to calcium CT scan testing. Adapted from reference 27, with permission

Table 7.5 Probability of a coronary event within 10 years calculated on the basis of results of EBCT[27]

Pretest probability of a coronary event within 10 years (%)	Probability of a coronary event within 10 years according to results of EBCT (%)	
	Calcium score ≥80	Calcium score <80
1.0	3.0	0.2
2.0	6.5	0.4
3.0	9.5	0.6
4.0	12.5	0.9
5.0	15.0	1.0
6.0	18.0	1.2
7.0	20.0	1.4
10.0	27.0	2.2
15.0	38.0	3.4
20.0	46.0	4.8

ommend calcium screening with CT of the general population[7].

CORONARY CALCIUM TO PREDICT SIGNIFICANT CORONARY OBSTRUCTIONS

The greater is the amount of calcium, the greater is the likelihood of a significant coronary obstruction, which, however, is not site specific. Calcium prediction for the presence of a significant coronary obstruction was established in 4394 patients (67% males), mean age 55.3 years, who all underwent coronary angiography with a prevalence of significant coronary artery disease of 52%[7]. The ability of the presence of calcium to predict a significant obstruction was high with a sensitivity of 93%, but with a low specificity of 45% and a predictive accuracy of 70% (Table 7.6). Rumberger *et al.* demonstrated that the low specificity can be addressed more comprehensively by comparing the calcium score and the degree of angiographic coronary lesion severity (Table 7.7)[31]. They performed a receiver-operating characteristic analysis to determine total calcium scores that provide 90% specificity for variable degrees of coronary stenoses. For example, an EBCT calcium score exceeding 27 gives 90% specificity for at least a 20% or greater risk of coronary stenosis. Haberl *et al.*[30] performed a comparative study between the calcium score in men

Table 7.6 Coronary calcium to predict significant (>50% diameter stenosis) coronary obstruction[7,30]

Subjects (n)	4394
Male (%)	67
Age mean (years)	55.3
Prevalence CAD (%)	52
Coronary calcium diagnostic performance	
Sensitivity (%)	93
Specificity (%)	45
Predictive accuracy (%)	70

Table 7.7 EBCT calcium score and 90% specificity of at least one coronary lesion being within the prescribed angiographic disease severity[31]

Angiographic disease severity (% diameter stenosis)	EBCT calcium score
≥20	27–88
≥30	89–127
≥40	128–166
≥50	167–370
≥70	≥370

and women and the outcome of invasive coronary angiography. They calculated the likelihood of the presence or absence of a significant coronary stenosis in relation to gender and age. The outcome is depicted in Figures 7.8 and 7.9. These data may be helpful to esti-

mate the likelihood of the presence of a significant coronary stenosis; they may also be helpful to adjust the sometimes difficult interpretation of a contrast-enhanced MSCT coronary angiogram of a patient with severe calcifications, which precludes accurate assess-

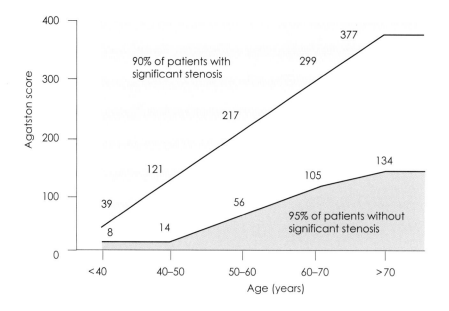

Figure 7.8 Calcium score to predict presence or absence of significant stenosis in men. From reference 30, with permission

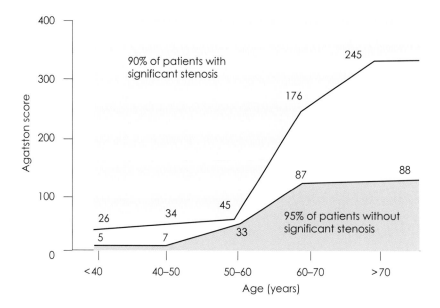

Figure 7.9 Calcium score to predict likelihood of presence or absence of significant stenosis in women. From reference 30, with permission

Table 7.8 Predictive value of calcium after diagnostic coronary angiography

	Detrano et al.[32] (422)	Keelan et al.[33] (288)
Age (years)	55±12	56±11
Follow-up (months)	30±13	71
Death/myocardial infarction (n)	13/8	22
CCS (Agatston)	≥75	≥10
Risk	6:1*	3.2*

*Compared to patients with lower calcium threshold or no presence of calcium; CCS, coronary calcium score

ment of the coronary lumen. However, one should keep in mind that there is not a direct one-to-one correlation between the site of detected coronary calcium and lumenal disease.

Coronary calcium to predict adverse events in patients who have undergone invasive coronary angiography

Symptomatic patients who have undergone invasive coronary angiography have been shown to be at high risk. However, the risk of these patients is further significantly increased by 3–6 times if coronary calcium is present compared to patients with no coronary calcium (Table 7.8)[32,33].

CONCLUSION

A high coronary calcium score, adjusted for age and sex, is a risk factor for adverse coronary events and may be helpful to remodify risk in individuals at intermediate risk in whom there is uncertainty about the institution of preventive measures[34].

REFERENCES

1. Rifkin RD, Parisi AF, Folland E. Coronary calcification in the diagnosis of coronary artery disease. Am J Cardiol 1979; 44: 141–7

2. McCarthy JH, Palmer FJ. Incidence and significance of coronary artery calcification. Br Heart J 1974; 36: 499–506

3. Rumberger JA, Simons DB, Fitzpatrick LA, et al. Coronary artery calcium area by electron-beam computed tomography and coronary atherosclerotic plaque area. A histopathologic correlative study. Circulation 1995; 92: 2157–62

4. Sangiorgi G, Rumberger JA, Severson A, et al. Arterial calcification and not lumen stenosis is highly correlated with atherosclerotic plaque burden in humans: a histologic study of 723 coronary artery segments using non-decalcifying methodology. J Am Coll Cardiol 1998; 89: 36–44

5. Mautner SL, Mautner GC, Froehlich J, et al. Coronary artery disease: prediction with in vitro electron beam CT. Radiology 1994; 192: 625–30

6. Simons DB, Schwartz RS, Edwards WD, et al. Noninvasive definition of anatomic coronary artery disease by ultrafast computed tomographic scanning: a quantitative pathologic comparison study. J Am Coll Cardiol 1992; 20: 1118–26

7. O'Rourke RA, Brundage BH, Froelicher VF, et al. American College of Cardiology/American Heart Association Expert Consensus document on electron-beam computed tomography for the diagnosis and prognosis of coronary artery disease. Circulation 2000; 102: 126–40

8. Schmermund A, Baumgart D, Gorge G, et al. Coronary artery calcium in acute coronary syndromes: a comparative study of electron-beam computed tomography, coronary angiography, and intracoronary ultrasound in survivors of acute myocardial infarction and unstable angina. Circulation 1997; 96: 1461–9

9. Schmermund A, Schwartz RS, Adamzik M, et al. Coronary atherosclerosis in unheralded sudden coronary death under age 50: histo-pathologic comparison with 'healthy' subjects dying out of hospital. Atherosclerosis 2001; 155: 499–508

10. Agatston AS, Janowitz WR, Hildner FJ, et al. Quantification of coronary artery calcium using ultra-

fast computed tomography. J Am Coll Cardiol 1990; 15: 827–32

11. Hoff JA, Chomka EV, Krainik AJ, et al. Age and gender distributions of coronary artery calcium detected by electron beam tomography in 35 246 adults. Am J Cardiol 2001; 87: 1335–9

12. Hoff JA, Quinn L, Sevrukov A, et al. The prevalence of coronary artery calcium among diabetic individuals without known coronary artery disease. J Am Coll Cardiol 2003; 41: 1008–12

13. Wong ND, Hsu JC, Detrano RC, et al. Coronary artery calcium evaluation by electron beam computed tomography and its relation to new cardiovascular events. Am J Cardiol 2000; 86: 495–8

14. Detrano RC, Doherty R, Wong ND, et al. Coronary calcium does not accurately predict near-term future coronary events in high-risk adults. Circulation 1999; 99: 2633–8

15. Raggi P, Cooil B, Callister TQ. Use of electron beam tomography data to develop models for prediction of hard coronary events. Am Heart J 2001; 141: 375–82

16. Raggi P, Callister TQ, Cooil B. Identification of patients at increased risk of first unheralded acute myocardial infarction by electron-beam computed tomography. Circulation 2000; 101: 850–5

17. Arad Y, Spadaro LA, Goodman K, Newstein D, Guerci AD. Prediction of coronary events with electron beam computed tomography. J Am Coll Cardiol 2000; 36: 1253–60

18. Kondos G, Hoff JA, Sevrukov A, et al. Electron-beam tomography coronary artery calcium and cardiac events. Circulation 2003; 107: 2571–6

19. Expert Panel on Detection, Evaluation and Treatment of High Blood Cholesterol in Adults. Executive summary of the Third Report of the National Cholesterol Education Program (NCEP). J Am Med Assoc 2001; 285: 2486–97

20. Pearson TA, Blair SN, Daniels SR, et al. AHA guidelines for primary prevention of cardiovascular disease and stroke: 2002 update; consensus panel guide to comprehensive risk reduction for adult patients without coronary or other atherosclerotic vascular diseases. Circulation 2002; 106: 388–91

21. Smith SC, Blair SN, Bonow RO, et al. AHA/ACC scientific statement: AHA/ACC guidelines for preventing heart attack and death in patients with atherosclerotic cardiovascular disease: 2001 update: a statement for healthcare professionals from the American Heart Association and the American College of Cardiology. Circulation 2001; 104: 1577–9

22. Jacobson TA, Griffiths GG, Varas C, et al. Impact of evidence-based 'clinical judgment' on the number of American adults requiring lipid-lowering therapy based on updated NHANES III data. National Health and Nutrition Examination Survey. Arch Intern Med 2000; 160: 1361–9

23. Greenland P, Smith SC Jr, Grundy SM. Improving coronary heart disease risk assessment in asymptomatic people: role of traditional risk factors and noninvasive cardiovascular tests. Circulation 2001; 104: 1863–7

24. Grundy SM. Primary prevention of coronary heart disease: integrating risk assessment with intervention. Circulation 1999; 100: 988–98

25. Smith SC Jr, Greenland P, Grundy SM. AHA Conference Proceedings. Prevention Conference V: Beyond secondary prevention: Identifying the high-risk patient for primary prevention: executive summary. American Heart Association. Circulation 2000; 101: 111–16

26. Greenland P, Abrams J, Aurigemma GP, et al. Prevention Conference V: Beyond secondary prevention: Identifying the high-risk patient for primary prevention: noninvasive tests of atherosclerotic burden: Writing Group III. Circulation 2000; 101: E16–22

27. Greenland P, Gaziano JM. Clinical practice. Selecting asymptomatic patients for coronary computed tomography or electrocardiographic exercise testing. N Engl J Med 2003; 349: 465–73

28. De Backer G, Ambrosioni E, Borch-Johnsen K, et al. European guidelines on cardiovascular disease prevention in clinical practice. Eur J Cardiovasc Prevent Rehabil 2003; 10: s1–10

29. Greenland P, LaBree L, Azen SP, et al. Coronary artery calcium score combined with Framingham score for risk prediction in asymptomatic individuals. J Am Med Assoc 2004; 291: 210–15

30. Haberl R, Becker A, Leber A, et al. Correlation of coronary calcification and angiographically documented stenoses in patients with suspected coronary artery disease: results of 1764 patients. J Am Coll Cardiol 2001; 37: 451–7

31. Rumberger JA, Brundage BH, Rader DJ, Kondos G. Electron beam computed tomographic coronary calcium scanning: a review and guidelines for use in asymptomatic persons. Mayo Clin Proc 1999; 74: 243–52

32. Detrano R, Hsiai T, Wang S. et al. Prognostic value of coronary calcification and angiographic stenoses in patients undergoing coronary angiography. J Am Coll Cardiol 1996; 27: 285–90

CHAPTER 8

Chronic total occlusion

Chronically occluded coronary lesions are present in 20–40% of patients with angiographically documented coronary artery disease[1,2]. They account for at least 10% of the target lesions of coronary angioplasty[3,4]. The success of percutaneous coronary intervention (PCI) is reported to be between 40% and over 80%[5,6], depending on certain characteristics of the occluded lesion and vessel. Characteristics associated with a high rate of failure to open the occluded vessel include age of occlusion > 3 months, length of occlusion more than 1.5 cm, stump missing, no tapered segment as an entry port and presence of bridging collaterals.

Multislice CT (MSCT) is able to detect a totally occluded lesion in about 95–100% of cases. MSCT-determined characteristics of the occlusion, such as degree of calcification or non-calcific tissue of the occluded segment, presence of calcium at the proximal entry port, length of the occluded vessel segment, or absence of a tapered segment as the entry port, may be helpful to predict the success rate of PCI. Mollet *et al.* performed a study investigating the predictive value of MSCT in addition to conventional coronary angiographic lesion characteristics to open chronically occluded coronary arteries in 45 patients[7]. They showed

that there were several MSCT predictors of failure to open chronically occluded coronary arteries (Table 8.1) (Figures 8.1 and 8.2).

In a multivariate analysis, it appeared that the absence of a tapered entry point as established by conventional coronary angiography was a predictor of

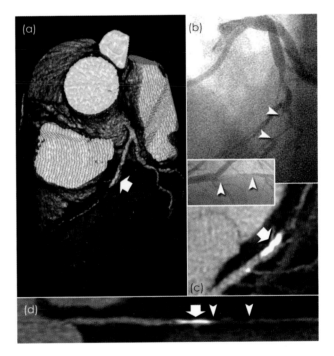

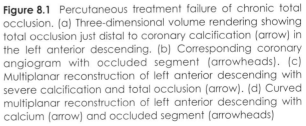

Figure 8.1 Percutaneous treatment failure of chronic total occlusion. (a) Three-dimensional volume rendering showing total occlusion just distal to coronary calcification (arrow) in the left anterior descending. (b) Corresponding coronary angiogram with occluded segment (arrowheads). (c) Multiplanar reconstruction of left anterior descending with severe calcification and total occlusion (arrow). (d) Curved multiplanar reconstruction of left anterior descending with calcium (arrow) and occluded segment (arrowheads)

Table 8.1 MSCT predictors of failure to open chronic total occlusion with percutaneous coronary intervention

Univariate MSCT predictors of failure
Occlusion length > 15 mm
Severe calcification of occluded segment
Stump morphology
Absence of tapered stump

Multivariate independent MSCT predictors of failure
Occlusion length > 15 mm
Severe calcification of occluded segment

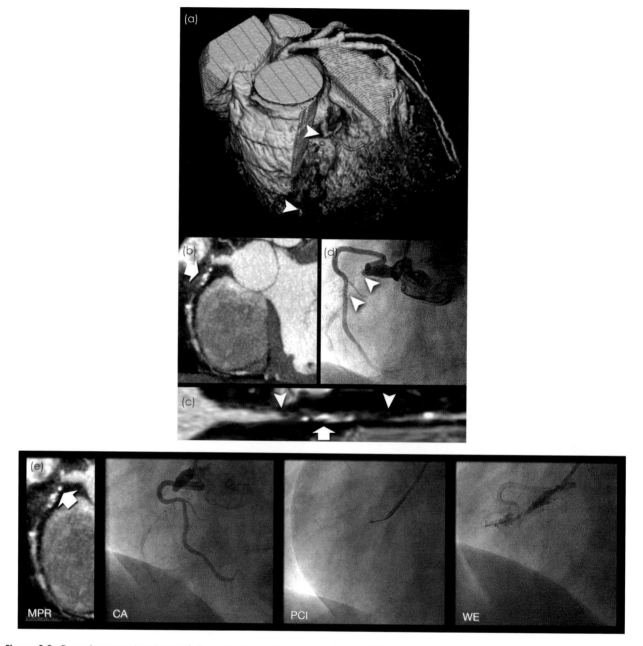

Figure 8.2 Percutaneous treatment failure of chronic total occlusion. (a) Volume-rendered image showing total occlusion of proximal right coronary artery (between arrowheads). The artery ends in a stump and origin of right ventricular branch. (b) Multiplanar reconstruction showing totally occluded proximal right coronary artery with occluded segment containing calcium (arrow). (c) Curved multiplanar reconstruction of occluded segment between arrowheads and calcification within occluded segment (arrow). (d) Corresponding invasive coronary angiogram showing total occlusion right coronary artery. (e) Failure of guide wire to cross the total occlusion and wire exit. Multiplanar reconstruction (MPR). Corresponding invasive coronary angiogram (CA), percutaneous coronary intervention (PCI): wire buckles at calcification in occluded segment and wire exit (WE)

failure. However, in addition the occlusion length > 15 mm and severe calcification both determined by MSCT were also independent predictors of procedural failure (Table 8.1) (Figure 8.3).

CONCLUSION

Non-invasive MSCT coronary angiographic predictors of failure of percutaneous coronary intervention to open

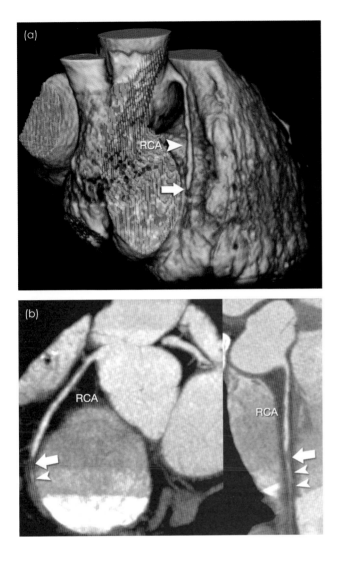

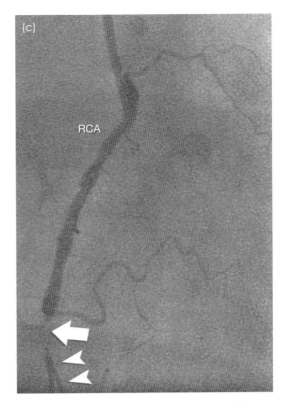

Figure 8.3 Successful percutaneous treatment of chronic total occlusion. (a) Volume-rendered image showing total occlusion of right coronary artery (RCA). (b) Multiplanar reconstruction and vessel view showing short occluded segment consisting of non-calcified tissue (arrow). The postoccluded distal part of the RCA is filled by collaterals (arrowheads). (c) Corresponding invasive coronary angiogram showing total occlusion of short segment with distal collateral filling of the RCA

chronically occluded coronary arteries are length of the occlusion and severe calcification of the occluded vessel segment. *A priori* knowledge before the PCI procedure may be helpful, and, for example, in case of severe calcification an intralumenal device or rotablation may be helpful.

REFERENCES

1. Baim DS, Ignatius EJ. Use of percutaneous translumenal coronary angioplasty: results of a current survey. Am J Cardiol 1988; 61: 3G–8G

2. Delacretaz E, Meier B. Therapeutic strategy with total coronary artery occlusions. Am J Cardiol 1997; 79: 185–7

3. Detre K, Holubkov R, Kelsey S, et al. Percutaneous transluminal coronary angioplasty in 1985–1986 and 1977–1981. The National Heart, Lung, and Blood Institute Registry. N Engl J Med 1988; 318: 265–70

4. Bell MR, Berger PB, Bresnahan JF, et al. Initial and long-term outcome of 354 patients after coronary balloon angioplasty of total coronary artery occlusions. Circulation 1992; 85: 1003–11

5. Puma JA, Sketch MH Jr, Tcheng JE, et al. Percutaneous revascularization of chronic coronary occlusions: an overview. J Am Coll Cardiol 1995; 26: 1–11

6. Olivari Z, Rubartelli P, Piscione F, et al. Immediate results and one-year clinical outcome after percutaneous coronary interventions in chronic total occlusions: data from a multicenter, prospective, observational study (TOAST-GISE). J Am Coll Cardiol 2003; 41: 1672–8

7. Mollet et al. Am J Cardiol 2004; accepted for publication

CHAPTER 9

Assessment of coronary stents

The number of patients with obstructive coronary artery disease who undergo coronary stent implantation is constantly increasing. Stent implantation has significantly reduced the occurrence of restenosis compared to balloon angioplasty, while drug-eluting stents have even further reduced the occurrence of in-stent restenosis. Obstructions within a coronary stent are caused by two processes: in-stent thrombosis and neointimal hyperplasia. Stent thrombosis can be acute (<48 h after stent implantation), subacute (2–30 days) or late (>30 days after stent implantation). The frequency of stent thrombotic occlusion is low and it occurs in about 1–1.5% of cases; however, its occurrence is clinically important because it is associated with a high mortality and morbidity. Neointimal hyperplasia occurs as a 'normal' healing process after stent implantation; however, in 15–25% of cases this may lead to in-stent restenosis defined as more than 50% diameter stenosis. Sometimes the neointimal hyperplasia is exuberant and total in-stent occlusion develops. The use of drug-eluting stents has significantly reduced the occurrence of in-stent restenosis due to neointimal hyperplasia to 5–9%.

Traditionally, in-stent restenosis has been assessed by invasive coronary angiography. A non-invasive alternative is the use of computed tomography (electron-beam (EBCT) or multislice (MSCT)); however, coronary stents have been notoriously difficult to assess by CT due to the stent-related high-density artifacts.

IN VITRO MSCT IMAGING OF CORONARY STENTS

Several types of stent manufactured from stainless steel were imaged after expansion in silicon tubes filled with contrast. The expanded stents were 3 and 4 mm in diameter. *In vitro* CT imaging showed that the stent struts appeared much larger than they actually were due to blooming artifacts. However, despite this, distinct patterns, unique to the stent type, were still visible, after *in vitro* MSCT imaging of larger stents with three-dimensional reconstruction. Unfortunately partial voluming artifacts and beam hardening resulted in a higher average CT density value of the stent lumen, which precluded in-stent assessment. Only in larger stents, with a diameter >4 mm, did there remain a small (1 mm) region of artifact-free lumen in the central stent lumen (Figure 9.1).

IN VIVO MSCT IMAGING OF CORONARY STENTS

Coronary stents are easily recognized on both non-enhanced and contrast-enhanced CT images because the

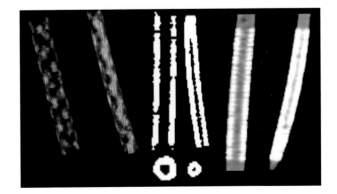

Figure 9.1 *In vitro* CT imaging of two CrossFlex™ stents, which are 2.5 and 4.0 mm in diameter. The stent pattern is visible. In the smaller stent due to significant 'blooming' artifact the lumen is not assessable whereas in the larger stent there is a small central artefact-free lumen

density of the stents is higher than that of any other tissue in or around the heart, including the contrast-enhanced lumen[1,2]. *In vivo* MSCT stent imaging suffers from the same in-stent imaging degrading artifacts as those seen in *in vitro* imaging. Again, the stent-related high-density artifacts enlarge the apparent size of the stent struts (Figure 9.2). This 'blooming effect' caused by a combination of partial voluming and beam harden-

ing is, in particular, quite disturbing in smaller-sized coronary stents with thick struts and relatively less disturbing in larger stents (> 4 mm in diameter) (Figure 9.3). In addition, cardiac motion artifacts, particularly with high heart rates, further reduce reliable assessment of coronary stents. The use of metal stents provides a major limitation for the clinical application of CT coronary angiography.

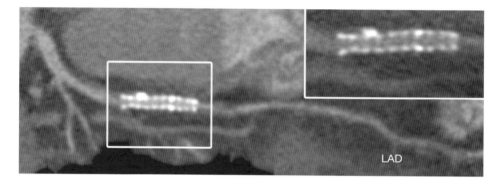

Figure 9.2 Curved multiplanar reconstruction of stent in mid-segment of left anterior descending (LAD). Note the apparent large size of the stent struts due to blooming artifacts. The in-stent lumen cannot be reliably assessed; however, the contrast enhancement of the distal LAD makes it highly likely that the stent is patent. The few bright 'dots' are calcific plaques; these are better visible in the insert

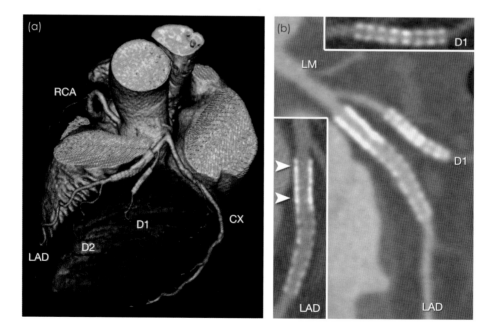

Figure 9.3 Volume-rendered image. (a) Stents in left anterior descending (LAD) and first diagonal branch (D1). (b) Multiplanar reconstruction. Stents in LAD: proximal stent has thick struts and distal stent thin struts. This causes there to be a significant difference in the apparent size of the stents. The stents in the LAD are 3.5 mm in diameter and allow crude assessment of the in-stent lumen (see insert). The stent in the D1 is 2.0 mm in diameter and the in-stent lumen is not assessable (see also insert). Both stents are patent because the vessels distal to the stents are clearly contrast enhanced. RCA, right coronary artery; D2, second diagonal branch; LCX, left circumflex

One way to circumvent the in-stent visualization problem is to utilize CT-flow studies to evaluate contrast enhancement distal to the stent for patency[3–6]. However, using the flow technique only severe, flow-limiting stenoses can be detected, and non-obstructive neointimal hyperplasia will not be noticed. Anatomical CT assessment of coronary stent lumen is useful and, in general, assessment of the patency of the stent is reliable. The 16-slice MSCT scanner permits assessment of neointimal hyperplasia and in-stent restenosis in larger stents (Figures 9.4–9.7). Kuboyama *et al.* studied 32 patients ±6 months after stent implantation in whom

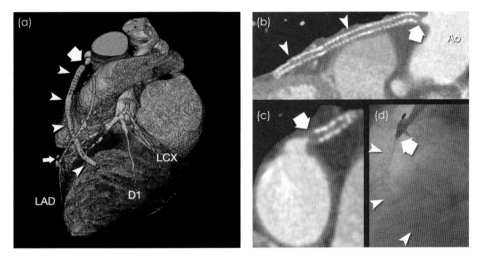

Figure 9.4 Volume-rendered image. (a) Stent in venous bypass graft. Very proximal (wide arrow) the bypass graft is occluded. The series of stents in the bypass are also occluded (arrowheads) and there is no bypass graft distal to the stent visible. A left internal mammary artery (LIMA) graft is visible with anastomosis at the left anterior descending (LAD) which cannot be assessed due to clip artifacts (arrow) and insufficient resolution. Multiplanar reconstruction of (b) venous bypass graft proximal occlusion (wide arrow) and occluded stents (arrowheads). (c) 'Blow up' of proximal venous bypass occlusion. The stump is contrast filled (open) and more distal without contrast (occlusion). (d) Corresponding invasive angiogram of the venous bypass graft confirming proximal occlusion (wide arrow). No distal filling of bypass graft. D1, first diagonal; LCX, left circumflex coronary artery; Ao, aorta

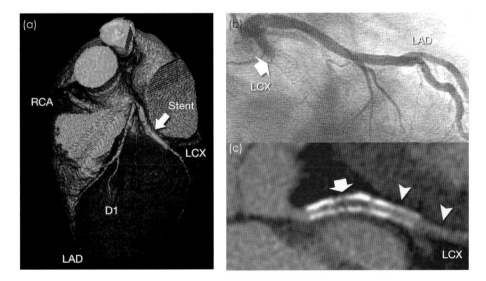

Figure 9.5 Volume-rendered image (a) showing stent in left circumflex (LCX) which is not patent. Multiplanar reconstruction (b) showing that the proximal part of the stent is patent, but more distally it is totally occluded (no contrast brightness in-stent lumen; arrow). (c) Distal part of stent and vessel is filled by collaterals (arrowheads). RCA, right coronary artery; LAD, left anterior descending; D1, first diagonal

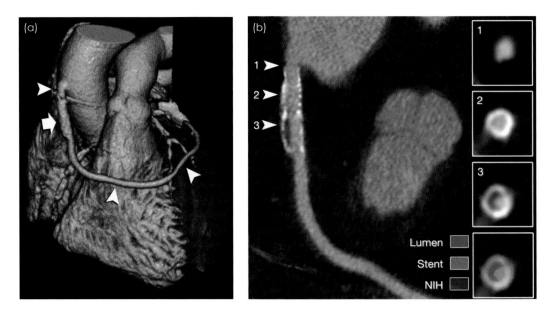

Figure 9.6 Volume-rendered image (a) showing stent in proximal venous bypass graft which is patent. Small lumen irregularities in bypass graft (arrowheads). (b) Curved multiplanar reconstruction showing (1) normal bypass lumen (see insert), (2) normal in-stent lumen (see insert), (3) neointimal hyperplasia (black rim), (insert) horse-shoe neointimal hyperplasia (NIH)

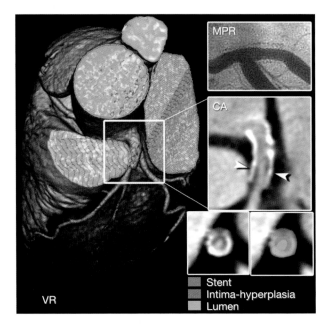

Figure 9.7 Volume-rendered image (VR) showing stent in left main artery. Multiplanar reconstruction (MPR) showing neointimal hyperplasia (dark rim of stent) in distal part of stent (arrowheads). Lower inserts show horse-shoe neointimal hyperplasia. Corresponding coronary angiogram (CA) showing stent struts and neointimal hyperplasia to be clearly visible

62 stents were implanted[7]. Fifty stents were evaluable for in-stent lumen assessment. Twelve stents were unevaluable due to thick stent struts, small stent size, severe calcification and motion artifacts. Sixteen-slice MSCT scanning detected 11 of the 12 in-stent restenoses (> 50% in-stent lumen diameter stenosis) and correctly detected the absence of restenosis in 27 of 38 stents; this resulted in a sensitivity of 92% and a specificity of 71%. Non-occlusive in-stent restenosis in smaller stents was not assessable. Post-stent implantation assessment with MSCT may be useful to assess the correct position of the stent, but unfortunately fails to identify the more subtle post-stent transplantation problems (Table 9.1) (Figures 9.8 and 9.9).

Requirements for reliable coronary stent imaging are MSCT scanners with thinner detectors to reduce partial volume effects, higher temporal resolution to reduce the motion artifacts, and possibly dedicated filtering of the acquired data to correct for high-density artifacts (Figure 9.10). However, the introduction of stents with a very thin strut, or biodegradable stents, would be the most effective means to improve stent imaging (Figure 9.11).

Table 9.1 MSCT coronary stent assessment

Possible
Patency/occlusion
Neointimal hyperplasia in large stents
In-stent restenosis in large stents
Stent position in ostial lesions
Stent overlap

Not possible
Neointimal hyperplasia in small stents
Tissue prolapse
Stent malapposition
Stent underexpansion

CONCLUSION

MSCT coronary stent imaging is useful to establish patency or complete stent obstruction. The latest 16-slice MSCT scanner permits evaluation of in-stent neointimal hyperplasia and in-stent restenosis. However, the spatial resolution needs to be improved to offer more reliable assessment of in-stent restenosis.

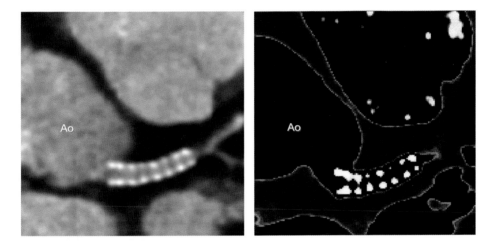

Figure 9.8 Multiplanar-reconstruction showing stent in left main artery. Part of the proximal stent is positioned in the left aortic sinus. Ao, aorta

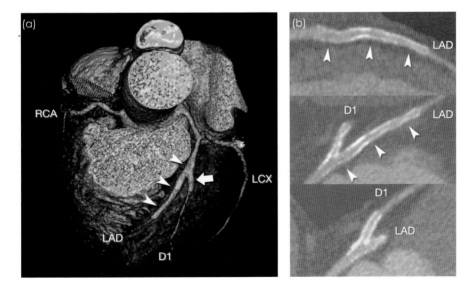

Figure 9.9 Volume-rendered image (a) showing bifurcation stent in left anterior descending (LAD) (arrowheads) first diagonal branch (D1) (arrow) using the 'crush' technique. Curved multiplanar reconstruction (b) showing 'crush' stent in left anterior descending and first diagonal branch. Distal stents in left anterior descending suggest stent under expansion (arrowheads). RCA, right coronary artery; LCX, left circumflex

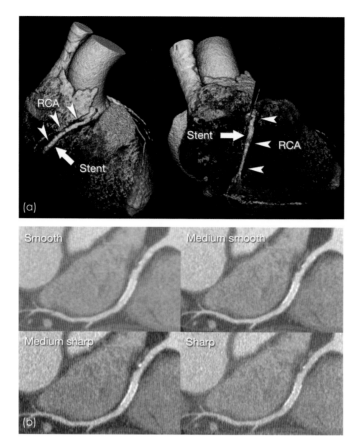

Figure 9.10 (a) Volume-rendered image of stent (arrow) in right coronary artery (RCA) (arrowheads). (b) Curved multiplanar reconstruction of stent in RCA; the stent is shown using various filters, which delineate the struts in different ways

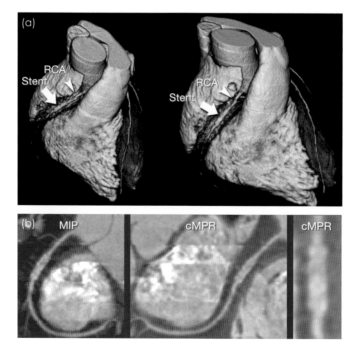

Figure 9.11 Volume-rendered image (a) showing stent in right coronary artery (RCA). (b) Maximum intensity projection (MIP) and curved multiplanar reconstruction (cMPR) of stent with very thin struts and almost no 'blooming' artifacts

REFERENCES

1. Nieman K, Cademartiri F, Raaijmakers R, et al. Noninvasive angiographic evaluation of coronary stents with multi-slice spiral computed tomography. Herz 2003; 28: 136–42

2. Mohlenkamp S, Pump H, Baumgart D, et al. Minimally invasive evaluation of coronary stents with electron beam computed tomography: in vivo and in vitro experience. Catheter Cardiovasc Interv 1999; 48: 39–47

3. Schmermund A, Haude M, Baumgart D, et al. Non-invasive assessment of coronary Palmaz-Schatz stents by contrast enhanced electron beam computed tomography. Eur Heart J 1996; 17: 1546–53

4. Pump H, Moehlenkamp S, Sehnert C, et al. Electron-beam CT in the noninvasive assessment of coronary stent patency. Acad Radiol 1998; 5: 858–62

5. Lu B, Dai RP, Bai H, et al. Detection and analysis of intracoronary artery stent after PTCA using contrast-enhanced three-dimensional electron beam tomography. J Invasive Cardiol 2000; 12: 1–6

6. Pump H, Moehlenkamp S, Sehnert CA, et al. Coronary arterial stent patency; assessment electron beam CT. Radiology 2000; 214: 447–52

7. Kuboyama et al. J Am Coll Cardiol 2004; 43: A364

CHAPTER 10

Coronary artery anomalies in the adult

Coronary artery anomalies are defined as abnormalities in the origin, course or distribution of coronary arteries. They are a rare form of congenital heart disease that affect approximately 1% of the population[1–6]. They are often the cause of sudden sport-related death in the young.

ANATOMY

The majority of the coronary anomalies have an ectopic origin of the coronary artery and frequently have associated congenital heart defects including mitral valve prolapse, bicuspid aortic valve, tetralogy of Fallot, transposition of the great vessels and aortic coarctation. Tetralogy of Fallot is associated with anomalous origin of the right coronary artery and transposition of the great arteries with a single coronary artery.

DIAGNOSIS OF CORONARY ANOMALIES

Traditionally the invasive technique of coronary angiography has been used to identify coronary anomalies[7,8]. However, it is sometimes difficult to visualize the abnormal course and, in particular, the course of an anomalous artery running between the aorta and pulmonary trunk may be difficult and requires specific projections and skillful interpretation. Three-dimensional coronary image reconstruction, from data obtained with magnetic resonance imaging (MRI) or computed tomography (CT), is extremely helpful and allows easy anatomical interpretation of the coronary anomalies. Schmid et al. investigated 20 patients with coronary anomalies[7]. The origin of all anomalous arteries and the exact course of 19 out of 20 patients was correctly iden-

tified (Table 10.1). The anatomical identification of coronary anomalies with MSCT is shown to be relatively easy; however, it remains difficult to identify which individuals are actually at high risk of sudden death.

MALIGNANT CORONARY ANOMALY

Sudden death is often associated with two anomalies: (1) the left main artery and right coronary artery arising from the right aortic sinus, with the anomalous left main coronary artery coursing between the aorta and pulmonary trunk; and (2) the left main coronary artery and right coronary artery originating from the left aortic sinus and the anomalous right coronary artery coursing between the aorta and pulmonary trunk (Figures 10.1–10.3).

Table 10.1 MSCT coronary anomalies[7]

Origin of coronary anomaly	Number of patients (n = 20)
Right-sided origin left main	9
Right-sided origin left CX	3
Right-sided origin LAD	1
Left-sided origin RCA	3
RCA from pulmonary artery	1
Coronary fistula to pulmonary artery	2
Fistula not correctly identified	1

CX, circumflex artery; LAD, left anterior descending artery; RCA, right coronary artery

(a)

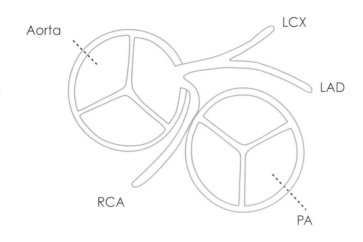

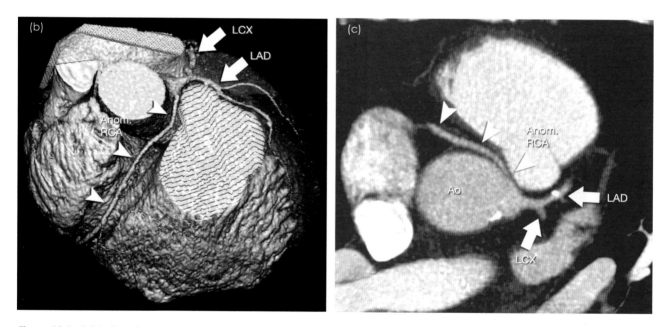

Figure 10.1 (a) Left main artery and right coronary artery (RCA) originating from left aortic sinus. (b) Volume-rendered image showing anomalous right coronary artery (Anom. RCA) originating from the left aortic sinus and coursing between the aorta (Ao) and pulmonary trunk (PA). (c) Cross-sectional image showing abnormal origin of right coronary artery from left aortic sinus and its course between aorta and pulmonary trunk. LAD, left anterior descending; LCX, left circumflex

BENIGN CORONARY ANOMALY

The majority of all coronary anomalies are benign and coincidental findings during coronary angiography. One of the most frequently occurring anomalies is the left circumflex artery and right coronary artery arising from the right aortic sinus. This anomaly is considered to be benign; however, awareness of this anomaly may be important during cardiac surgery to institute appropriate myocardial protection (Figures 10.4 and 10.5).

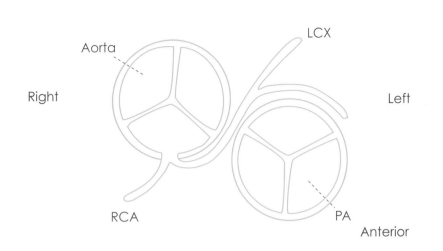

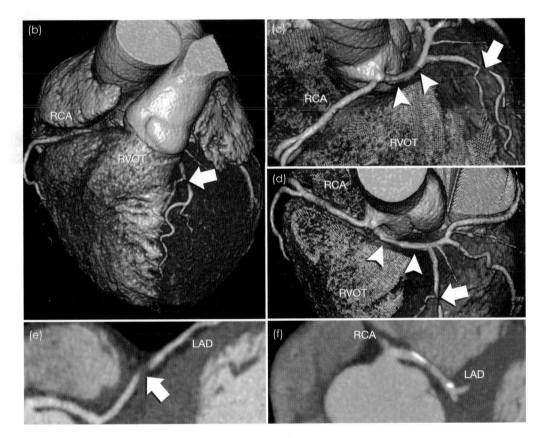

Figure 10.2 (a) Left main artery and right coronary artery (RCA) arising from the right aortic sinus. (b)–(d) Volume-rendered images showing left main and right coronary artery arising from the right aortic sinus. The anomalous left main coronary artery courses between the aorta and pulmonary trunk (arrowheads). Note severe lesion in the left anterior descending (LAD) (arrow). (e) and (f) Multiplanar reconstructions showing left main coronary artery originating from right aortic sinus and coursing between the aorta and pulmonary trunk. Note severe lesion in left anterior descending (arrow). RVOT, right ventricle outflow track

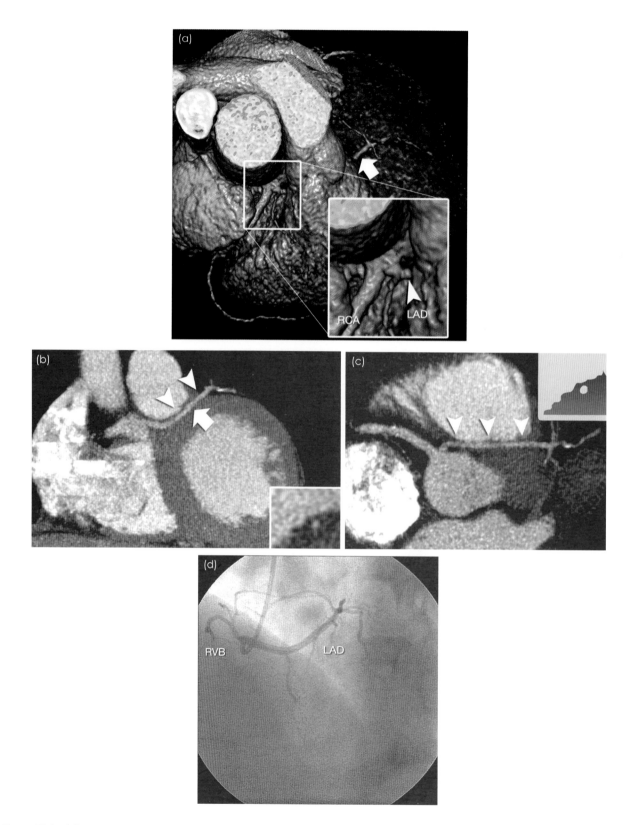

Figure 10.3 (a) Volume-rendered image showing the left main coronary artery originating from the right aortic sinus and running between the aorta and pulmonary artery to the anterior left ventricle wall (arrow). (b) and (c) Multiplanar reconstructions showing the abnormal origin and course of the left main running between the aorta and pulmonary artery (arrowheads). (d) Corresponding invasive coronary angiogram. RVB, right ventricular branch; LAD, left anterior descending

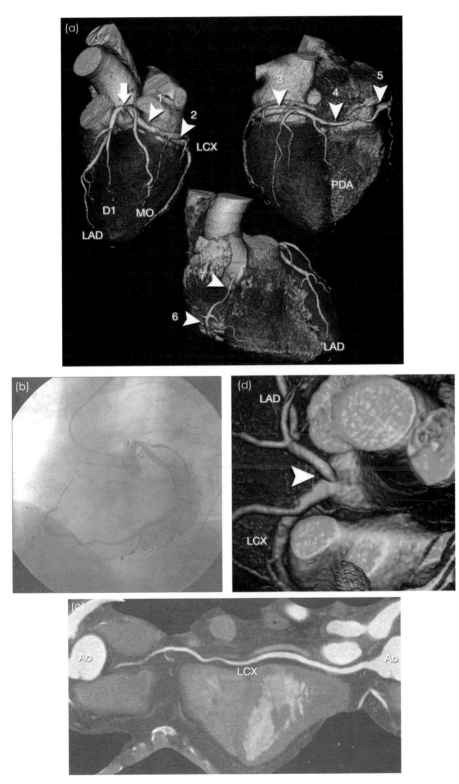

Figure 10.4 (a) Volume-rendered image demonstrating normal left anterior descending (LAD) and large left circumflex (LCX) (1) and (2) running over the diaphragm (3) to branch into a posterior descending artery (PDA) and running (4) and (5) further over the heart to end almost at the right aortic sinus (6) and (7). There is no right coronary artery. (b) Corresponding invasive coronary angiogram. (c) Curved multiplanar reconstruction demonstrating the course of the left circumflex from left aortic sinus to almost the right aortic sinus. (d) Volume-rendered image showing a separate ostium of the LAD and LCX. D1, first diagonal; MO, marginal obtuse; Ao, aorta

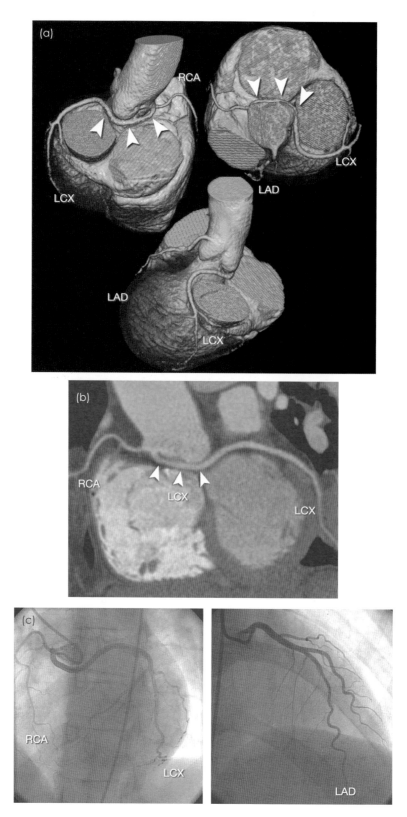

Figure 10.5 (a) Volume-rendered image showing left circumflex (LCX) originating from the right aortic sinus and running between the left atrium and aortic into the left atrioventricular groove (arrowheads). (b) Multiplanar reconstruction showing the left circumflex originating from the right aortic cusp and running to the left atrioventricular groove (arrowheads). (c) Corresponding invasive coronary angiogram. LAD, left anterior descending; RCA, right coronary artery

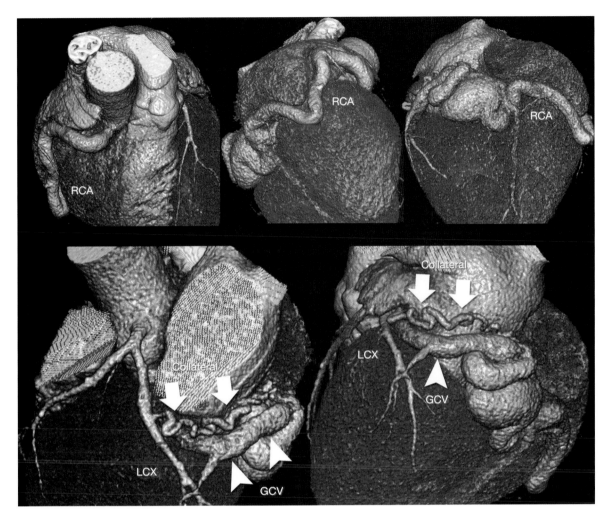

Figure 10.6 Volume-rendered images showing an enormous fistula from the right coronary artery (RCA) ending in the coronary sinus and a smaller fistula running from the left circumflex (LCX) to the coronary sinus. GCV, great cardiac vein

CORONARY ARTERY FISTULAE

Coronary artery fistulae usually involve the right coronary artery. The usual site of termination is in one or more low-pressure structures: right or left atrium, right ventricle, coronary sinus, pulmonary artery or superior vena cava. The fistulae appear as dilated (sometimes huge) tortuous communications between a coronary artery and low-pressure cardiac structure (Figures 10.6 and 10.7).

CONCLUSION

Non-invasive CT scanning of the heart allows correct identification of coronary anomalies and three-dimen-sional reconstruction allows precise insight into the course of the coronary anomalies to identify whether these anomalies are malignant or benign.

REFERENCES

1. Topaz O, DeMarchena EJ, Perin E, et al. Anomalous coronary arteries: angiographic findings in 80 patients. Int J Cardiol 1992; 34: 129–38

2. Yamanaka O, Hobbs RE. Coronary artery anomalies in 126 595 patients undergoing coronary arteriography. Cathet Cardiovasc Diagn 1990; 21: 28–40

3. Taylor AJ, Rogan KM, Virmani E. Sudden cardiac death associated with isolated congenital coronary artery anomalies. J Am Coll Cardiol 1992; 20: 640–7

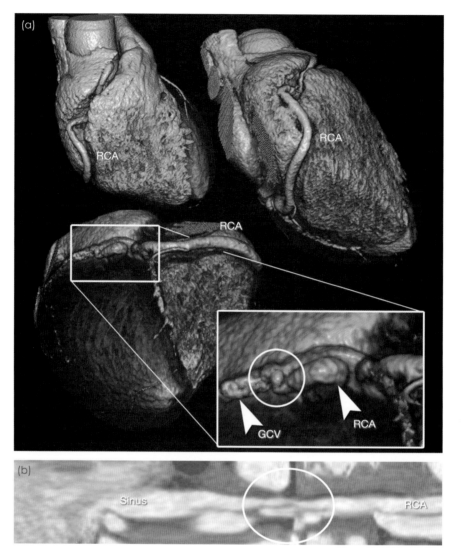

Figure 10.7 (a) Volume-rendered image showing fistula between right coronary artery (RCA) and great cardiac vein (GCV). The right coronary artery is large and tortuous. The insert shows the connection between the right coronary artery and great cardiac vein (O). (b) Curved multiplanar reconstruction detailed image of the connection between right coronary artery and great cardiac vein

4. Maron BJ, Shirani J, Poliac LC, et al. Sudden death in young competitive athletes. Clinical, demographic, and pathological profiles. J Am Med Assoc 1996; 276: 199–204

5. Roberts WC. Major anomalies of coronary arterial origin seen in adulthood. Am Heart J 1986; 111: 941–63

6. Taylor AJ, Virmani R. Coronary artery anomalies. In Crawford MH, DiMarco JP, eds. Cardiology. Chapter 10. London: Mosby, 2001

7. Schmid M, Ropers D, Pohle K, et al. Detection of coronary anomalies by submillimeter 16-slice spiral computed tomography. J Am Coll Cardiol 2004; (Suppl): abstr 312

8. Ropers D, Moshage W, Daniel WG, et al. Visualization of coronary artery anomalies and their anatomic course by contrast-enhanced electron beam tomography and three-dimensional reconstruction. Am J Cardiol 2001; 87: 193–7

CHAPTER 11

Assessment of collateral circulation

Coronary collaterals are said to be present when part of a coronary artery is visible beyond the site of an occlusion or severe stenosis with thrombolysis in myocardial infarction (TIMI) flow 1 or 2.

Collaterals can be classified as intra- and intercoronary. They may be epicardiac in location, when they course over the surface of the heart, or transmural, when they transverse the myocardium such as the interventricular septum. The most commonly encountered collateral pathways are:

(1)   Left to right transseptal or periapical from the anterior descending to the posterior descending or vice versa;

(2)   Left to right from the distal circumflex to the distal right coronary artery;

(3)   Intracoronary collaterals around an obstruction.

The collateral circulation can be visualized using MSCT coronary angiography (Figures 11.1 and 11.2). In particular, well-developed coronary collaterals, which course over the surface of the heart, that may exist in the case of a totally occluded coronary artery with complete opacification of the distally occluded coronary segments, and is associated with almost normal left ventricular wall motion, can be visualized.

The less well-developed intercoronary collaterals and the small intracoronary collaterals usually are not visible with CT imaging.

CONCLUSION

Only very well-developed collaterals can be visualized with CT coronary angiography.

BIBLIOGRAPHY

Levin DC. Pathways and functional significance of the coronary collateral circulation. Circulation 1974; 50: 831–6

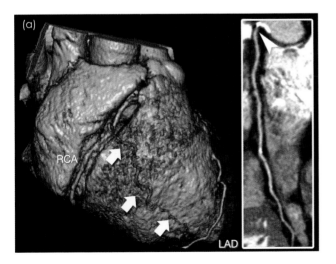

Figure 11.1 (a) Volume-rendered image (left panel, right lateral view) showing a collateral artery (Coll.) (arrows) running from the left anterior descending coronary artery (LAD) towards the right coronary artery (RCA). The curved multiplanar reconstructed image (right panel) shows a severely calcified ostial occlusion of the right coronary artery. (b) Volume-rendered image (left panel, right lateral view) after successful percutaneous treatment of the total occlusion. The collateral can no longer be visualized after stenting. The curved multiplanar reconstructed image (right panel) shows the stent at the ostium of the right coronary artery and an increased vessel diameter compared to pretreatment (a). (c) Corresponding invasive angiogram. A selective injection in the left coronary artery confirms the presence of a collateral artery (arrowheads) arising from the left anterior descending coronary artery and collateral filling of the occluded right coronary artery (arrow) *(see overleaf)*

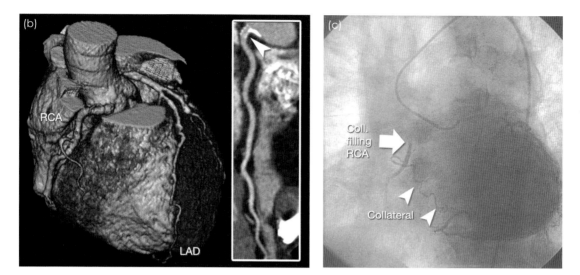

Figure 11.1 *Continued*

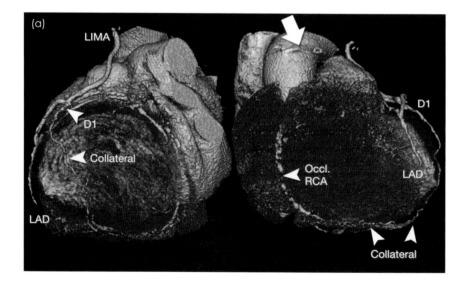

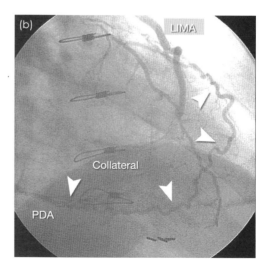

Figure 11.2 (a) Volume-rendered images showing a collateral artery arising from the first diagonal branch (D1) towards the posterior descending coronary artery (PDA). This patient has a patent left internal mammary artery (LIMA) supplying the left anterior descending coronary artery (LAD), an occluded venous graft (arrow) and an occluded right coronary artery (Occl. RCA). (b) Corresponding invasive angiogram confirming the presence of the collateral artery (arrowheads) arising from the diagonal branch towards the posterior descending coronary artery and the patent left internal mammary artery

CHAPTER 12

Coronary bypass graft imaging

CORONARY BYPASS GRAFT SURGERY

One of the therapeutic options in patients with symptomatic coronary artery disease is coronary artery bypass graft (CABG) surgery. Depleted myocardium is reperfused by a surgically inserted vessel distal to the obstruction. Various material can be used, but most grafts are either saphenous vein grafts or internal mammary artery grafts (Figure 12.1). Saphenous veins are free grafts that require surgical anastomosis to the (ascending) aorta. The internal mammary arteries can also be used for grafting, and have a much higher long-term patency rate. Mobilization of the internal mammary artery is a delicate procedure and involves clipping of the intercostal side-branches.

Single attached grafts are only inserted into a single coronary artery, while sequential grafts are inserted into a sequence of coronary artery branches. Up to 10% of grafts become occluded during the perioperative period[1]. After 10 years occlusion rates of 59% and 17% have been reported for venous and arterial grafts, respectively[2]. Of patients who undergo bypass surgery, 40% will experience recurrence of symptoms within 6 years, and 25% of bypass grafts are found to be occluded at follow-up 5 years after surgery[3–6]. Patients who have undergone CABG in the past will be older, present with co-morbidity and have a higher prevalence of valvular heart disease and ventricular dysfunction. Compared with non-CABG patients they will have a higher incidence of complications during invasive proce-

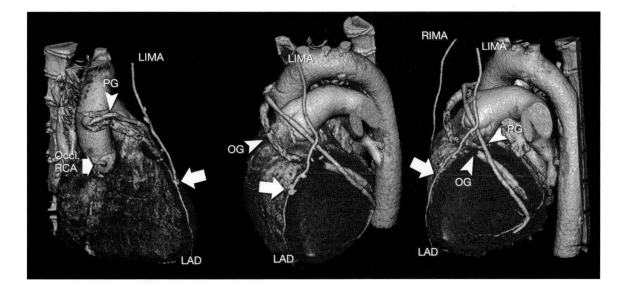

Figure 12.1 Volume-rendered images showing a patent left internal mammary artery (LIMA) inserted into the left anterior descending coronary artery (LAD). Anastomosis of the LIMA on the LAD (arrow). An occluded venous graft (OG arrowheads) with several stents, a redo patent venous graft (PG arrowhead) inserted into a marginal branch and an occluded right coronary artery (Occl. RCA short arrow) are also visualized. The right internal mammary artery (RIMA) is *in situ*

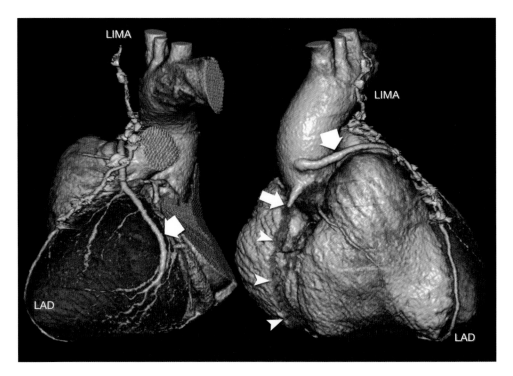

Figure 12.2 Volume-rendered images. The left internal mammary artery (LIMA) is almost completely obscured by artifacts caused by the surgical clips. Venous grafts are often better visualized owing to the absence of surgical clips. A patent venous graft inserted on the marginal branches (thick arrow) and an occluded venous graft (thin arrow) towards the occluded right coronary artery (arrowheads) are well visualized. LAD, left anterior descending coronary artery

dures, including cardiac catheterizations, and may therefore benefit more from non-invasive coronary angiography.

GRAFT IMAGING

Because of their large diameter, limited calcification and relative immobility, bypass grafts, and particularly saphenous vein grafts, are well visualized by CT (Figure 12.1). In order to image the entire graft an extended scan range is required. Surgical radiopaque material such as sutures, clips and markers may cause artifacts and interfere with the interpretation of the grafts (Figure 12.2). While the radiopaque material at the site of the anastomosis of a venous graft is useful to guide future catheterization procedures, the indicator at the site of the graft's orifice may hinder evaluation of the proximal grafts using CT. Grafts that run across the anterior surface of the heart may be close to the sternal wires. If metal-containing material is used to clip side-branches of the graft, evaluation may become difficult.

Using four-slice CT the proximal part of the mammary artery is usually not included. A 4×1.0-mm detector collimation complete acquisition would require a much longer scan time than any patient can hold his breath. To image the entire mammary artery, either a wider detector collimation is selected or a protocol with a caudocranial scan direction that permits respiration near the end of the acquisition. Using 16-slice technology neither of these concessions are needed, and the entire graft can be acquired at high resolution during a manageable breath-hold time.

CLINICAL PERFORMANCE AND LIMITATIONS

With respect to the evaluation of patients who underwent bypass surgery a number of aspects can be included. Complete occlusion of a graft is possible and the utilization of electron-beam angiography to detect the patency of bypass grafts has been reported since as early as 1986. Sequential studies during dynamic contrast enhancement as well as CT angiography have been explored with electron-beam CT[7-12], with a sensitivity and specificity of 75–100% and 86–100%, respectively, to detect total graft occlusion. Single-slice spiral CT flow measurements have also been used to determine graft patency with a sensitivity and specificity of 86–92% and 100%[13,14]. However, severely stenosed but patent bypass grafts remained undetected, the proximal and distal anastomoses were not evaluated and approximately 15% of the bypass grafts were not evaluable.

Current spiral CT technology allows more accurate evaluation of graft patency with a sensitivity approaching 100% in both arterial and venous grafts without exclusion of grafts due to insufficient image quality[15-18] (Table 12.1) (Figures 12.3 and 12.4). In sequential grafts, each segment can be evaluated separately[17]. Detection of graft stenosis without occlusion has been shown with four-slice and even better with 16-slice scanners[15,17,18] (Figure 12.3). In the published studies to date, not all graft segments were assessable with respect to non-complete lumenal narrowing and only small numbers of lesions were included in each study.

Ischemic symptoms in patients after bypass surgery can be caused by obstruction of bypass grafts, or by progression of disease in the native coronary arteries. Therefore, evaluation cannot be limited to the bypass grafts but should also include the coronary arteries. In theory the evaluation of the coronary arteries should be similar to that in patients without a surgical history. However, in reality the majority of these post-surgical patients are older, and have diffuse coronary artery disease and more advanced atherosclerosis with more severe calcification[17]. Under such circumstances detection of significant lumenal narrowing can be challenging (Figure 12.4). Particularly in post-surgical patients, functional information is essential to determine whether an angiographic lesion is hemodynamically significant or not. In addition, some investigators have reported that up to 10% of venous grafts become occluded shortly after the surgical procedure, sometimes without obvious symptoms[1]. Therefore, functional non-invasive information may be required to determine whether the finding of an occluded bypass graft is responsible for the patient's symptoms.

Advantages of MSCT are that it shows ventricular wall thinning after a myocardial infarction and allows for non-invasive three-dimensional assessment of the (resting) ventricular function. In addition to the fact that there is no need for intra-arterial introduction of catheters, there is also no need for localization and intubation of the bypass grafts or coronary arteries. Information regarding the atherosclerotic status of both the target coronary artery and potential arterial graft may be helpful when re-intervention is considered.

LIMITATIONS

The presence of opaque material, such as vascular clips, sternal wires and graft orifice indicators, complicates evaluation of coronary grafts. Angiographic evaluation after surgical coronary intervention should include assessment of the native coronary arteries, which tends to be more difficult compared to that in non-CABG patients. Coronary flow and myocardial perfusion

Table 12.1 Diagnostic performance of spiral CT after bypass surgery. Data in parenthese are number of graft segments in sequential grafts

| | CT slices | | Graft types | | Total occlusion | | | Stenosis (50–99%) | | |
| | | | | | Exclusion | Sensitivity | Specificity | Exclusion | Sensitivity | Specificity |
Study	(n)	n	Arterial	Venous	(%)	(%)	(%)	(%)	(%)	(%)
Ropers et al.[15]	4	65	182		—	97	98	38	75	92
Yoo et al.[16]	4	42	70	55	NR	98	100	—	—	—
Nieman et al.*[17]	4	24	18 (26)	23 (60)	8 16	100 95	97 94	9 5	60 83	88 90
Anders et al.[18]	16	34	11	50	—	100	100	16	80	90

*Analysis of graft segments by two observers. Only venous grafts evaluated for non-complete obstruction; NR, not reported

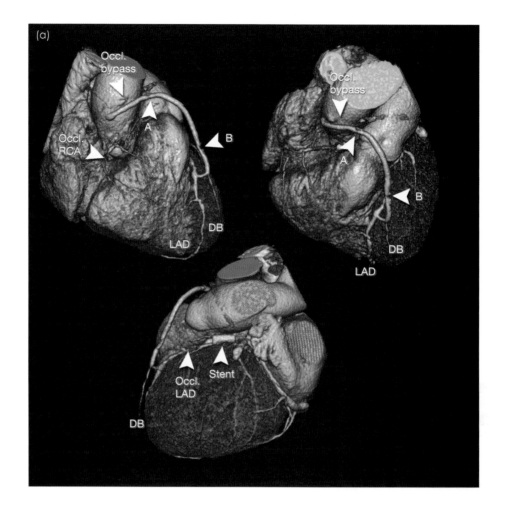

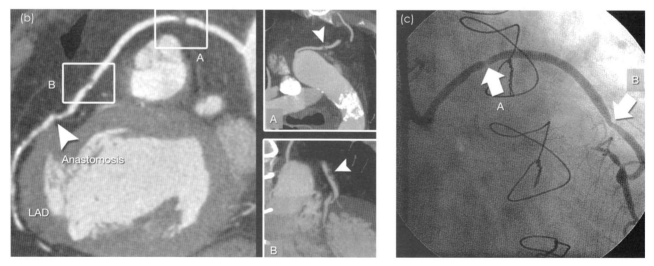

Figure 12.3 (a) Volume-rendered images showing an occluded venous graft towards the circumflex coronary artery, and a patent venous graft inserted into a diagonal branch (DB) and into the left anterior descending coronary artery (LAD). Two lesions are present in the patent graft (A) and (B) arrowheads. The occlusion of the left anterior descending and a proximal stent are shown in the lower image. (b) Curved multiplanar-reconstructed image showing the lesions in the graft (boxes (A) and (B)) as well as the anastomosis and distal filling of the left anterior descending coronary artery. The right panels are maximum-intensity projected images showing the proximal (A) and distal (B) lesions in more detail. (c) An invasive angiogram confirmed the presence of two significant lesions (A) and (B) in the venous graft

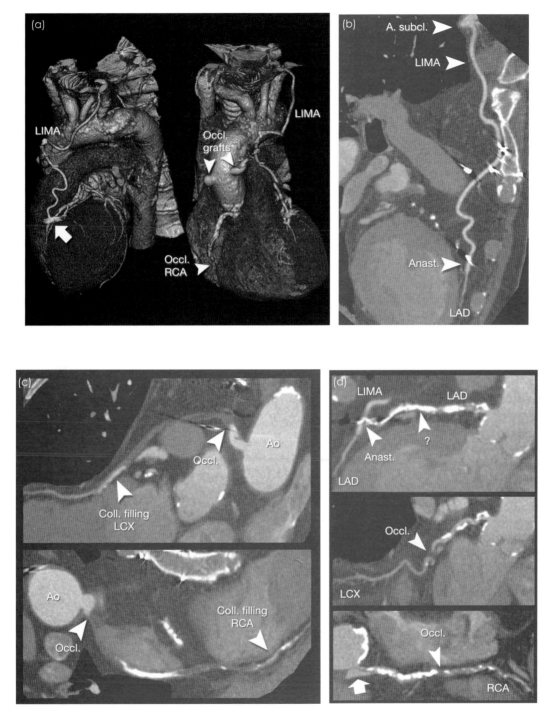

Figure 12.4 (a) Volume-rendered images showing a patent left internal mammary artery (LIMA) inserted into the left anterior descending coronary artery (LAD). However, the presence of a surgical clip precludes reliable visualization of the anastomosis (arrow). Two occluded (Occl.) venous grafts are visualized as well as an occluded right coronary artery (RCA) (arrowheads). (b) Curved multiplanar-reconstructed image showing the left internal mammary artery and distal filling of the left anterior descending coronary artery. (c) Curved multiplanar-reconstructed images of the occluded venous grafts (arrowheads) and collateral (Coll.) filling of the circumflex coronary artery (LCX) (top panel) and right coronary artery (bottom panel). (d) Curved multiplanar-reconstructed images of the left anterior descending coronary artery (upper panel), circumflex coronary artery (middle panel) and right coronary artery (lower panel). The occlusions within the non-calcified areas of the left circumflex and right coronary artery are clearly visualized, whereas extensive calcification of the left anterior descending precludes reliable evaluation of the coronary lumen (question mark). The arrow (lower panel) indicates the presence of an aneurysm of the right coronary artery. Ao, aorta; A. Subcl., arteria subclavia; Anast, anastomosis

cannot be evaluated, but are of great importance in the evaluation of post-CABG patients.

CONCLUSION

CT scanning of venous bypass grafts and arterial grafts is associated with a high sensitivity and specificity to detect significant obstructions. The assessment of patency of the grafts has a sensitivity of almost 100%. Remaining problems are the assessment of, in particular, graft anastomoses. Comprehensive post-bypass surgery evaluation should also include the assessment of the native coronary arteries, which is difficult in these patients owing to the diffuse nature of the disease, and the frequent presence of severe calcifications.

REFERENCES

1. Bryan AJ, Angelini GD. The biology of saphenous vein occlusion: etiology and stratagies for prevention. Curr Opin Cardiol 1994; 9: 641–9

2. Barner HB, Standeven JW, Reese J. Twelve-year experience with internal mammary artery for coronary artery bypass. J Thorac Cardiovasc Surg 1985; 90: 668–75

3. Cameron A, Davis KB, Rogers WJ. Recurrence of angina after coronary artery bypass surgery: predictors and progression (CASS Registry). J Am Coll Cardiol 1995; 26: 895–9

4. Fitzgibbon GM, Kafka HP, Leach AJ, et al. Coronary bypass graft fate and patient outcome: angiographic follow-up of 5065 grafts related to survival and reoperation in 1388 patients during 25 years. J Am Coll Cardiol 1996; 28: 616–26

5. Christenson JT, Simonet F, Schmuziger M. Sequential vein bypass grafting: tactics and long-term results. Cardiovasc Surg 1998; 6: 389–97

6. Dion R, Glineur D, Derouck D, et al. Complementary saphenous grafting: long-term follow-up. J Thorac Cardiovasc Surg 2001; 122: 296–304

7. Bateman TM, Gray RJ, Whiting JS, et al. Cine computed tomographic evaluation of aortocoronary bypass graft patency. J Am Coll Cardiol 1986; 8: 693–8

8. Bateman TM, Gray RJ, Whiting JS, et al. Prospective evaluation of ultrafast cardiac computed tomography for determination of coronary bypass graft patency. Circulation 1987; 75: 1018–24

9. Stanford W, Brundage BH, MacMillan R, et al. Sensitivity and specificity of assessing coronary bypass graft patency with ultrafast computed tomography: results of a multicenter study. J Am Coll Cardiol 1988; 12: 1–7

10. Achenbach S, Moshage W, Ropers D. Non-invasive, three-dimensional visualization of coronary artery bypass grafts by electron beam tomography. Am J Cardiol 1997; 79: 856–61

11. Ha JW, Cho SY, Shim WH, et al. Non-invasive evaluation of coronary artery bypass graft patency using three-dimensional angiography obtained with contrast-enhanced electron beam CT. Am J Roentgenol 1999; 172: 1055–9

12. Lu B, Dai RP, Jing BL, et al. Evaluation of coronary artery bypass graft patency using three-dimensional reconstruction and flow study on electron beam tomography. J Comput Assist Tomogr 2000; 24: 663–70

13. Engelmann MG, von Smekal A, Knez A, et al. Accuracy of spiral computed tomography for identifying arterial and venous coronary graft patency. Am J Cardiol 1997; 80: 569–74

14. Tello R, Costello P, Ecker C, Hartnell G. Spiral CT evaluation of coronary artery bypass graft patency. J Comput Assist Tomogr 1993; 17: 253–9

15. Ropers D, Ulzheimer S, Wenkel E, et al. Investigation of aortocoronary artery bypass grafts by multislice computed tomography with electrocardiographic-gated image reconstruction. Am J Cardiol 2001; 88: 792–5

16. Yoo KJ, Choi D, Choi BW, et al. The comparison of the graft patency after coronary artery bypass grafting using coronary angiography and multislice computed tomography. Eur J Cardiothorac Surg 2003; 24: 86–91

17. Nieman K, Pattynama PMT, Rensing BJ, et al. CT angiographic evaluation of post-CABG patients: assessment of grafts and coronary arteries. Radiology 2003; 229: 749–56

18. Anders K, Baum U, Ropers D, et al. Non-invasive investigation of coronary artery bypass grafts using multi-detector spiral computed tomography with sub-millimeter collimation. Radiology 2003; 229(Suppl) RSNA abstract p.584

CHAPTER 13

Cardiac masses, intracardiac thrombi and pericardial abnormalities

Cardiac masses, intracardiac thrombi and pericardial abnormalities are infrequently occurring abnormalities, that can be identified by CT cardiac imaging[1–4].

INTRACARDIAC TUMORS (Figures 13.1–13.4)

Atrial myxomas account for 50% of intracardiac tumors. They are usually located in the left atrium attached to the atrial septum at the fossa ovalis and are often pedunculated. Rhabdomyomas, fibromas and lipomas are less frequently occurring benign cardiac tumors. Metastatic tumors most frequently arise from melanomas and lung and breast carcinomas. Intracavitary tumor masses appear as filling defects within the contrast-filled heart chambers, or are seen as filling deformities of the cardiac cavities.

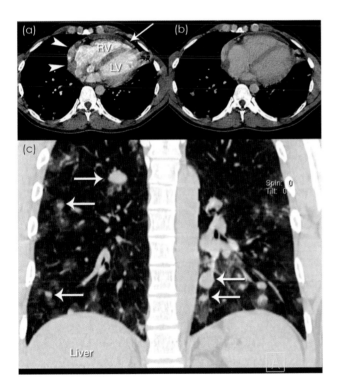

Figure 13.1 Right atrial angiosarcoma. (a) Wall thickening of right atrium (arrowheads) and pericardial effusion (arrow). (b) Delayed phase of enhancement. (c) Long metastases (arrows). RV, right ventricle; LV, left ventricle

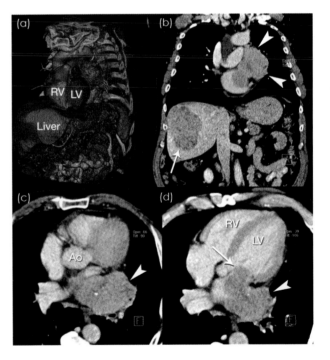

Figure 13.2 Cardiac carcinoid tumor. Volume-rendered image of thorax and upper abdomen. (a) Carcinoid tumor in right liver lobe and left atrium. (b) Carcinoid tumor in liver (arrow) and large tumor in left atrium (arrowheads). (c) and (d) Large carcinoid tumor in left atrium (arrowhead), almost totally occupying the left atrium, and bulging through mitral valve (arrow). RV, right ventricle; LV, left ventricle; Ao, aorta

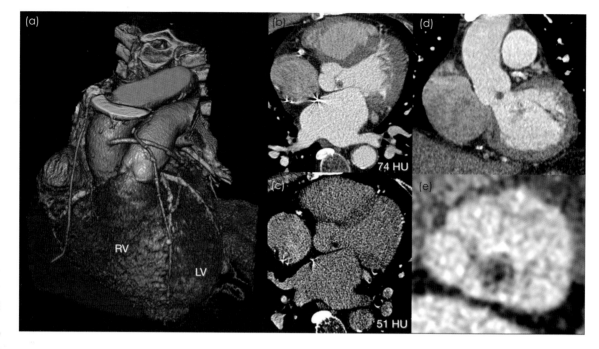

Figure 13.3 Aortic valve fibroelastoma. (a) Volume-rendered image of the heart. Venous bypass graft with anastomosis on left circumflex artery and left internal mammary artery with anastomosis on left anterior descending. (b), (c) and (d) Round filling defect in left aortic sinus attached to aortic valve. (e) Enlargement showing filling defect. RV, right ventricle; LV, left ventricle

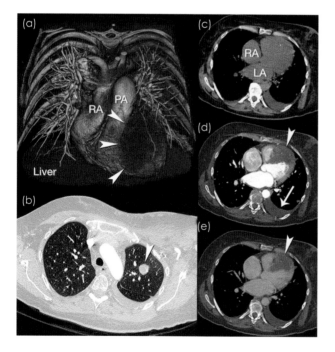

Figure 13.4 Breast carcinoma with metastases in heart. (a) Volume-rendered image with metastasis of right and left ventricle (arrowheads). (b) Lung metastasis (arrowhead). (c)–(e) Enormous filling defect in right and left ventricle (arrowheads) and pleural effusion (arrows). RA, right atrium; PA, pulmonary artery

INTRACARDIAC THROMBI (Figures 13.5–13.7)

Intracardiac thrombi are usually seen as filling defects within the contrast-filled cardiac chambers. In the left ventricle they are usually located at the site of an infarcted myocardium most frequently in the apex of the left ventricle following a large anterior wall myocardial infarction. Usually the thrombus is mural, but sometimes may be pedunculated. Long-standing thrombi can be calcified. The left atrial appendage is another frequently occurring site of intracardiac thrombus, in particular in patients with mitral stenosis and atrial fibrillation.

PERICARDIAL ABNORMALITIES (Figures 13.8 and 13.9)

The pericardium can usually be seen as a 1–2-mm thick, linear low-density structure lying between the mediastinal fat ventrally and the epicardial fat dorsally. Constrictive pericarditis causes a thickening of the pericardium, which may be localized or diffuse and is often associated with tuberculosis, tumor infiltration or

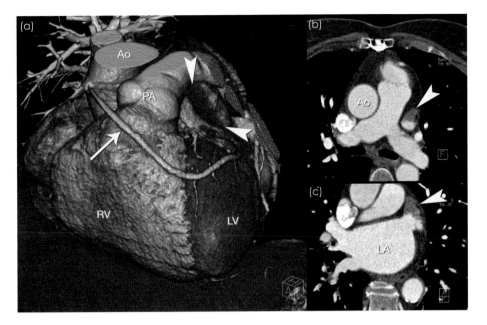

Figure 13.5 Left atrial thrombus. (a) Volume-rendered image showing venous bypass graft running from the aorta (Ao) to left anterior descending, first diagonal and left circumflex (arrow). Left atrial appendage (arrowheads). (b) and (c) Filling defect of part of left atrial appendage (arrowheads). RV, right ventricle; LV, left ventricle; Ao, aorta; PA, pulmonary artery; LA, left atrium

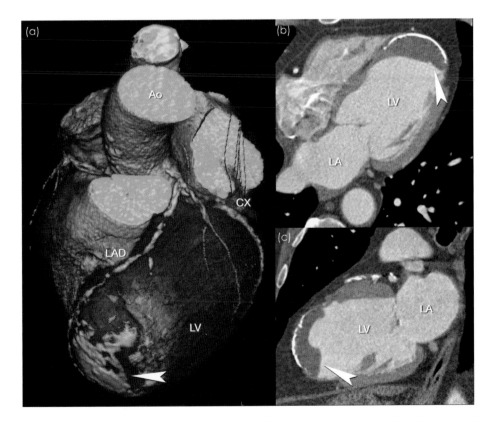

Figure 13.6 (a) Volume-rendered image of left coronary artery with extensive coronary calcifications. The left ventricular apex is enlarged and calcified (arrowhead). (b) and (c) Extensive filling defect of apex of the left ventricle (LV) caused by organized thrombus (arrowheads). Note severe calcification of apex. LAD, left anterior descending; LCX, left circumflex; Ao, aorta; LA, left atrium

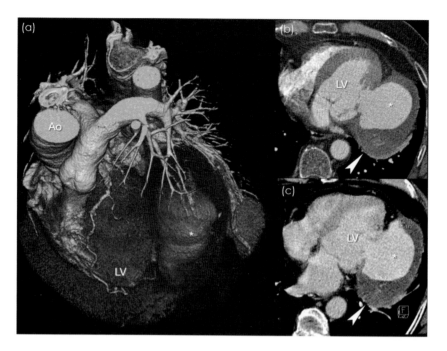

Figure 13.7 Left ventricular false aneurysm (*). (a) Volume-rendered image. (b) and (c) Large false aneurysm with 'short neck'. The aneurysm is largely 'filled' by organized thrombotic material (arrowhead). LV, left ventricle; Ao, aorta

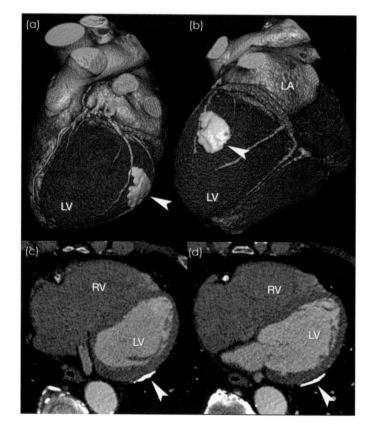

Figure 13.8 Pericardial calcification. (a) and (b) Volume-rendered images with areas of calcification in the pericardium (arrowheads). (c) and (d) Pericardial calcification (arrowheads). LV, left ventricle; LA, left atrium; RV, right ventricle; LV, left ventricle

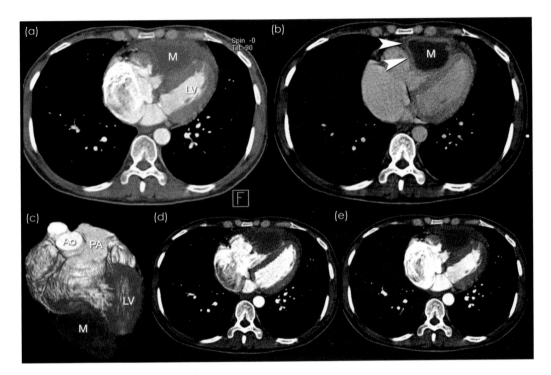

Figure 13.9 Pericardial abscess (M). (a)–(e) Pericardial non-contrast-filled abscess with surrounding rim of contrast enhancement (M) (arrowheads). The right ventricle is compressed. (c) Volume-rendered image showing abscess (M) involving pericardium and compression of right ventricle. LV, left ventricle; M, abscess (mass); Ao, aorta; PA, pulmonary artery

infections. The thickened pericardium may cause constriction of the myocardium which hampers diastolic left ventricular filling. This should be differentiated from restrictive cardiomyopathy where the pericardium is normal.

Pericardial effusion, diffusely located, small in amounts or as massive fluid accumulation, is most readily seen on CT imaging.

Pericardial cysts are unusual but readily identifiable by CT because they are filled with low-density fluid that has an attenuation value (HU) similar to water. Benign and malignant pericardial tumors are rare.

CONCLUSION

Multislice CT (MSCT) is a useful, non-invasive technique for the evaluation of intracardiac masses, intracardiac thrombi and pericardial disease.

REFERENCES

1. Bleiweis MS, Georgiou D, Brundage BH. Detection of intracardiac masses by ultrafast computed tomography. Am J Card Imaging 1994; 8: 63–8

2. Georgiou D, Bleiweis MS, Brundage BH. Ultrafast computed tomography in the diagnosis of diseases of great vessels. Am J Card Imaging 1993; 7: 120–7

3. Galvin JR, Gingrich RD, Hoffman E, et al. Ultrafast computed tomography of the chest. Radiol Clin North Am 1994; 32: 775–93

4. Lipton MJ, Higgins CB, Boyd DP. Computed tomography of the heart: evaluation of anatomy and function. J Am Coll Cardiol 1985; 5(Suppl 1): 55S–69S

CHAPTER 14

The emergency department

Patients presenting with (acute) chest pain at an emergency department can pose a difficult diagnostic problem, in particular, when they have no or non-specific electrocardiographic abnormalities and no history of previous coronary artery disease. Specific cardiac enzyme levels to detect or exclude coronary abnormalities require 6–12 h of observation, and a less time-consuming diagnostic method to detect coronary abnormalities would be highly desirable. In this respect CT coronary calcium can play a role in the diagnostic work-up of patients admitted to an emergency department presenting with acute chest pain. The presence of coronary calcification assessed by CT may increase the likelihood that coronary artery disease is the cause of the acute chest pain, and should require further in-hospital diagnostic work-up, whereas in patients with absence of calcium the likelihood of a flow-limiting coronary stenosis is very low, and discharge of the patient may be safe (Figures 14.1–14.3).

Laudon et al. examined 100 patients with angina-like chest pain presenting at the emergency department who all underwent electron-beam CT (EBCT) to identify coronary calcium[1]. The EBCT findings were compared with other cardiac evaluation findings in the patients, such as treadmill stress testing, radionuclide testing, dobutamine echo stress testing and coronary angiography. The scan was positive if the calcium was more than 0. Only younger patients were studied: men between 30 and 55 years of age and women between 40 and 65 years of age. The sensitivity of a positive calcium scan was 100% (95% confidence interval (CI) 77–100%) when compared with the positive cardiac evaluation findings. The specificity was 63% (95% CI 54–75%). The negative predictive value of 100% suggests that patients without the presence of calcium are at extremely low risk of an adverse coronary event.

The value of the calcium scan to predict cardiac death and non-fatal myocardial infarction in patients presenting with chest pain at an emergency department was assessed by McLaughlin et al. and Georgiou et al[2,3]. Both studies indicated that a positive calcium scan was associated with an increased risk of adverse coronary events (Table 14.1). Furthermore, it appeared that a higher calcium score was associated with a higher annualized event rate (Figure 14.4) and that after adjustment for age and gender, the relative risk significantly increased in patients with calcium scores in the third and fourth quartiles (Figure 14.5). Furthermore, a negative

Table 14.1 Value of calcium to predict cardiac death and non-fatal myocardial infarction (MI) in patients presenting at emergency department

Calcium scan	McLaughlin et al.[2] (n = 134)		Georgiou et al.[3] (n = 192)	
	n	Event rate at 30 days (%)	n	Event rate at 50 ± 10 months (%)
Negative	48	0	76	0
Positive	86	4.4 (non-fatal MI n = 4)	116	15.6 (cardiac deaths n = 11, non-fatal MI n = 19)

Annualized rates of cardiovascular events: death, MI, coronary artery bypass graft, percutaneous translumenal coronary angioplasty, hospitalization for angina and ischemic stroke[3]

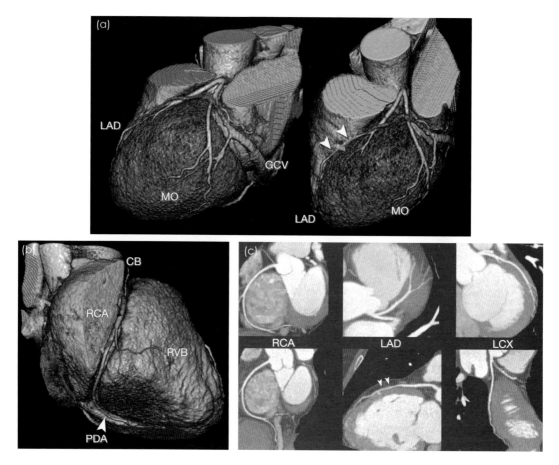

Figure 14.1 Patient with atypical chest pain. (a) Left coronary artery absence of coronary calcium and no coronary artery lumen abnormalities. Left anterior descending (LAD) runs in the myocardium (arrowheads). (b) Right coronary artery (RCA) with no abnormalities. (c) Multiplanar reconstruction showing intramyocardial course of left anterior descending (arrows). MO, marginal obtuse; GCV, great cardiac vein; RVB, right ventricular branch; PDA, posterior descending artery (arrowhead); LCX, left circumflex

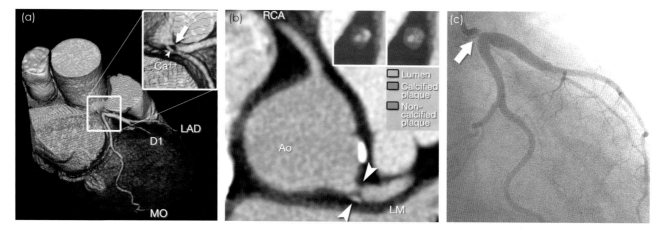

Figure 14.2 Young female patient presenting with chest pain and non-specific T wave abnormalities. (a) Severe stenosis (large arrow) and calcification (arrowhead) of left main artery. (b) Cross-sectional image of left main showing stenosis (between arrowheads). Right upper panels show orthogonal projection at site of left main stenosis. (c) Corresponding invasive coronary angiography demonstrating severe left main stenosis (arrow). LAD, left anterior descending; D1, first diagonal; MO, marginal obtuse; LM, left main; Ao, aorta; RCA, right coronary artery

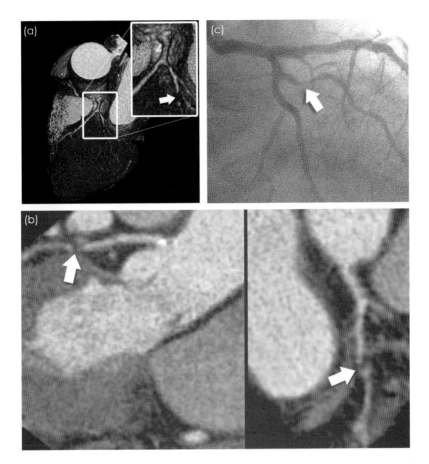

Figure 14.3 Patient with typical chest pain and ST segment depressions. (a) Left coronary artery. Left main and left anterior descending are normal. Left circumflex has a severe lesion at bifurcation (arrow) of obtuse marginal branch. (b) Multiplanar reconstruction. Non-calcific severe lesion at bifurcation (arrows). Calcium is present in the proximal part of the artery (bright spot). (c) Corresponding invasive coronary angiography with lesion in obtuse marginal branch (arrow)

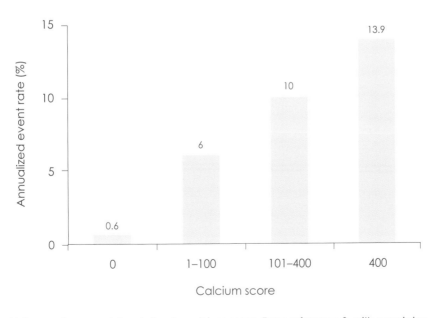

Figure 14.4 Relative risk for cardiac events in relation to calcium score. From reference 3, with permission

calcium score was associated with a very low risk of adverse coronary events.

To date, no studies are available that have assessed the value of CT coronary angiography in combination with CT coronary calcium quantification in the setting of the evaluation of acute chest pain in an emergency department. However, it seems reasonable to assume that the combined information would be clinically relevant (Figures 14.6 and 14.7).

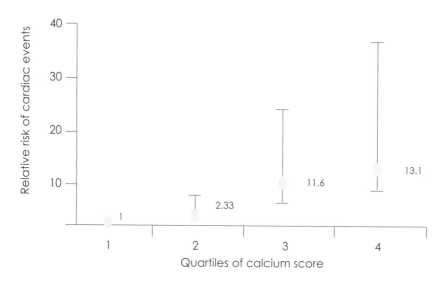

Figure 14.5 Relative risk for cardiac vascular events using age- and gender-adjusted quartiles. Confidence intervals (95%) are presented for each quartile. From reference 3, with permission

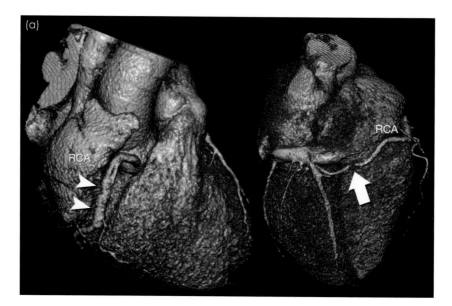

Figure 14.6 Patient with chest pain and no electrocardiographic abnormalities. Previously the patient underwent a stent implantation in the right coronary artery (RCA). (a) Left panel shows stent in right coronary artery. Right panel shows severe lesion in distal right coronary artery. (b) Multiplanar reconstructions. Left panel shows no calcification. Mid-right coronary artery shows a stent. Distal right coronary artery shows a non-calcific severe lesion (arrow). Insert is an orthogonal view of the lesion. Right panel shows severe lesion in distal right coronary artery (arrow). (c) Corresponding invasive diagnostic angiography showing severe lesion (arrow)

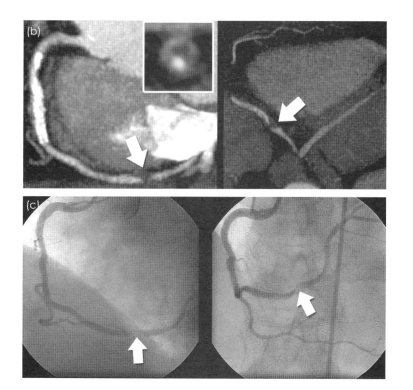

Figure 14.6 *Continued.*

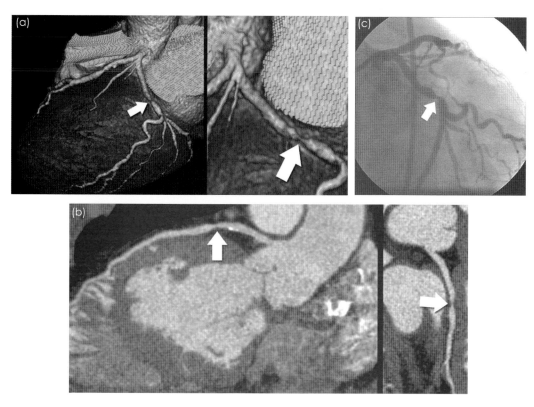

Figure 14.7 Patient with atypical chest pain and no electrocardiographic abnormalities. (a) Left coronary artery showing normal left anterior descending and a severe lesion (arrows) of the left circumflex. (b) Multiplanar reconstruction showing non-calcific significant lesion in left circumflex (arrows). (c) Corresponding diagnostic invasive angiography showing severe lesion in left circumflex

CONCLUSION

Middle-aged individuals admitted with chest pain to an emergency department who have a negative calcium scan can be safely discharged, obviating the need for further provocative testing. The predictive value of a positive calcium scan is low, and therefore further testing is required in individuals with a positive calcium scan.

REFERENCES

1. Laudon DA, Vukov LF, Breen JF, et al. Use of electron-beam computed tomography in the evaluation of chest pain patients in the emergency department. Ann Emerg Med 1999; 33: 15–21

2. McLaughlin VV, Balogh T, Rich S. Utility of electron beam computed tomography to stratify patients presenting to the emergency room with chest pain. Am J Cardiol 1999; 84: 327–8

3. Georgiou D, Budoff MJ, Kaufer E, et al. Screening patients with chest pain in the emergency department using electron beam tomography: a follow-up study. J Am Coll Cardiol 2001; 38: 105–10

CHAPTER 15

The great thoracic vessels

Aortic aneurysms and dissections are associated with significant morbidity and mortality, and quick precise delineation of the underlying pathoanatomy is highly desirable and helpful for more favorable surgical management of these often critically ill patients. For many years invasive contrast angiography has been the reference standard, but contrast angiography is limited because it shows only the lumen of the vessel and lacks the significant additional information of cross-sectional images and subsequent three-dimensional reconstructed images that are provided by CT angiography[1,2].

AORTIC ANEURYSM (Figures 15.1 and 15.2)

An aortic aneurysm is an abnormal dilatation of the aorta, to at least 50% larger than normal.

The majority of aortic aneurysms are caused by atherosclerosis, while other causes include Marfan syndrome, cystic media necrosis, trauma and post-stenotic dilatation of infectious mycotic disease.

Aneurysms are classified according to their shape, fusiform or saccular, and can be classified as true or false. A true aneurysm has an intact aortic wall, is usually

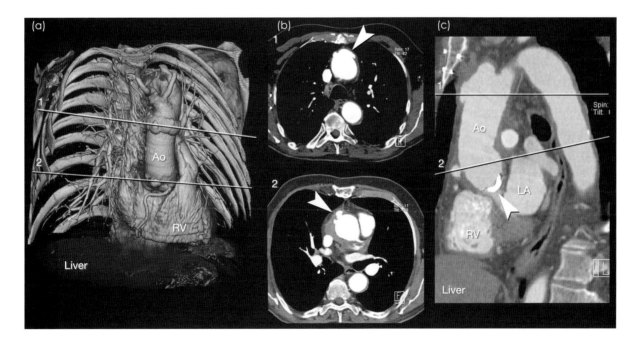

Figure 15.1 False aneurysms of the ascending aorta (Ao). (a) Volume-rendered image. (1) and (2) refer to cross-sectional images, (1) and (2) in (b), and show two false aneurysms (arrowhead). (c) Reformatted reconstruction with calcified aortic valve (arrowhead). RV, right ventricle; LA, left atrium

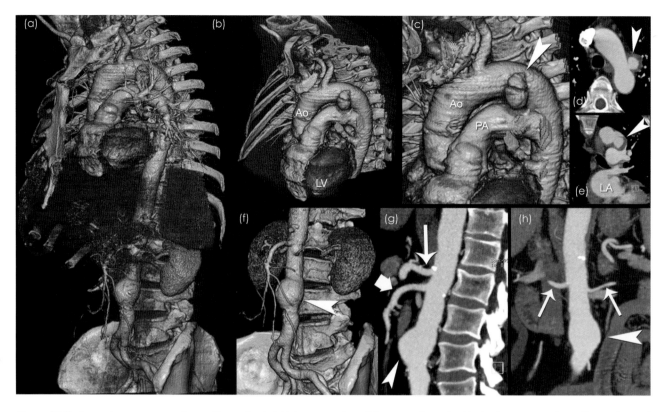

Figure 15.2 Saccular aneurysm in aortic arch. (a) Volume-rendered image of aorta (Ao). Aneurysm at aortic arch and abdominal aorta (f)–(h). (b)–(d) Enlargements of aortic arch saccular aneurysm (arrowhead). (d) and (e) Contrast-enhanced multiplanar reconstruction of aortic arch with saccular aneurysm (arrowheads). (f)–(g), (h) Fusiform aneurysm in abdominal aorta (arrowhead), below level of celiac trunk (thin arrow) and superior mesenteric artery (thick arrow). Fusiform aneurysm below renal arteries (arrows). PA, pulmonary artery; LV, left ventricle; LA, left atrium

fusiform and is associated with atherosclerosis. A false aneurysm is caused by a disruption of the wall, is usually saccular and is associated with infection or atherosclerosis. Both fusiform and saccular aneurysms may contain a thrombus. Aortic aneurysms have the tendency to expand.

AORTIC DISSECTION (Figures 15.3 and 15.4)

Aortic dissection is caused by a small tear in the intima, which propagates by dissecting the intima from the tunica media and the adventitia thus creating two channels: a false channel and a true channel[1,2]. The false channel is often large, may either become thrombosed or remain patent and may end blindly or re-enter the true lumen through a distal tear. Dissections can be classified according to the De Bakey classification or the Stanford classification. A dissection involving both the ascending and descending thoracic aorta is classified as

De Bakey type I, if only the aorta ascendens is involved as De Bakey type II and if only the descending aorta is involved as De Bakey type III. The Stanford classification is based upon prognostic grounds. Type A involves dissection of the ascending aorta. These dissections have a poor prognosis and require immediate surgery. Type B involves dissections of the descending aorta, which have a better prognosis. Computed tomography of an aortic dissection has typical features:

(1)   Intimal flap separating the true and false lumen;

(2)   Contrast enhancement occurs first in the true lumen and later in the false lumen;

(3)   Inward displacement of intimal calcification by the false lumen;

(4)   Often presence of thrombosis within the false lumen;

(5)   Thickening of the aortic wall.

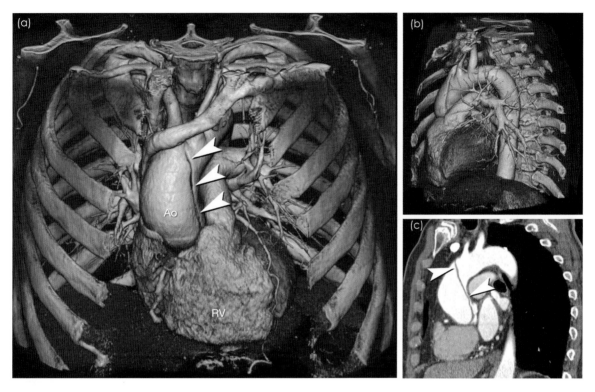

Figure 15.3 (a) and (b) Volume-rendered images of aorta showing dissection (arrowheads) in the ascending aorta (Ao) during diastole. (c) Multiplanar reconstruction (during diastole) showing dissection in the ascending aorta (arrowheads). RV, right ventricle

INTRAMURAL HEMORRHAGE OF THE AORTA

Intramural hemorrhage can be described as a dissection without an initial tear which is now considered to be an imminent precursor of aortic dissection. Aortic intramural hematoma is caused by rupture of the vasovasorum in the medial wall layers[3]. CT allows identification of an intramural hemorrhage as a non-enhancing circular or crescent-shaped localized wall thickening, with the high-density appearance of a fresh hematoma and absence of an intimal flap or tear. Thrombosis is identified by a multilayered appearance.

PENETRATING AORTIC ULCER

A penetrating aortic ulcer is an atheromatous plaque that ulcerates and disrupts the internal elastic lamina, and penetrates the aortic media and beyond[4]. On CT a penetrating aortic ulcer is diagnosed as a contrast-material filled out-pouching in the aorta in the absence of a dissection flap or false lumen.

CONGENITAL AORTIC DISEASE (Figures 15.5–15.8)

Patients with Marfan syndrome may show cardiovascular involvement with progressive aortic-root dilatation, and subsequent aortic insufficiency, dissection or rupture. Coarctation of the aorta is associated with a localized narrowing of the aorta just distal to the ductus arteriosus. This anomaly is often associated with a bicuspid aortic valve. Both anomalies can be accurately identified by CT angiography.

PULMONARY EMBOLI (Figure 15.9)

Pulmonary emboli are seen as filling defects in the contrast-enhanced pulmonary arteries, and spiral CT has a high accuracy in identifying pulmonary emboli. CT scanning is excellent for the diagnosis of a central large pulmonary embolism but is less reliable for clinically important smaller pulmonary emboli in the peripheral pulmonary arteries[5,6].

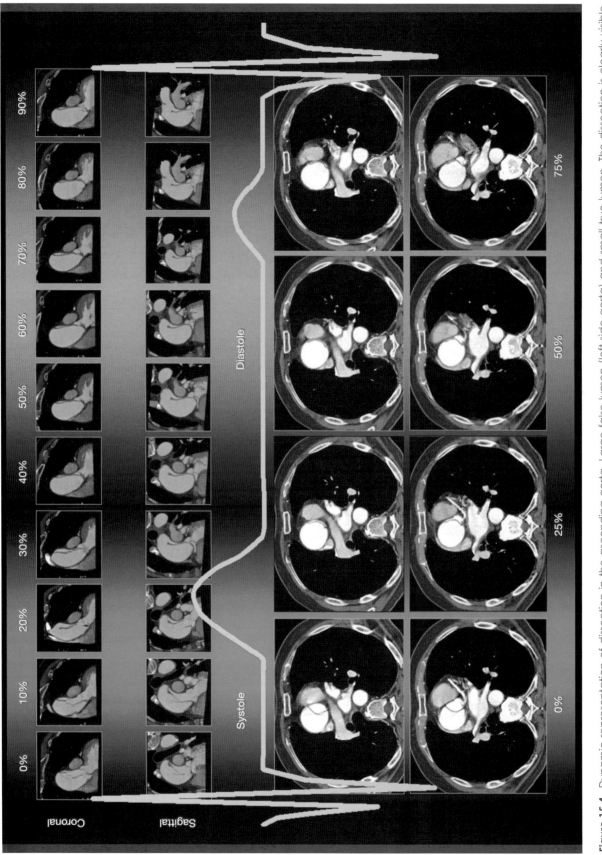

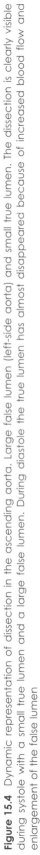

Figure 15.4 Dynamic representation of dissection in the ascending aorta. Large false lumen (left-side aorta) and small true lumen. The dissection is clearly visible during systole with a small true lumen and a large false lumen. During diastole the true lumen has almost disappeared because of increased blood flow and enlargement of the false lumen

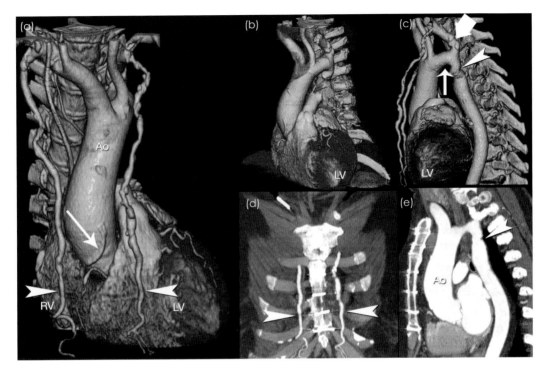

Figure 15.5 Coarctation aorta. (a) Volume-rendered image of an aorta (Ao) with a scar at the root of the aorta ascending (arrow) owing to a previous surgical incision (valve replacement and surgical repair of coarctation). The left internal mammary artery (LIMA) and right internal mammary artery (RIMA) are shown (arrowheads). (b) and (c) Volume-rendered images of aorta showing coarctation of aorta with tubular aortic arch (arrow) and residual narrowing after surgical repair (arrowhead). Left subclavian artery with calcifications is shown (wide arrow). (d) Maximum-intensity projection of LIMA and RIMA (arrowheads). (e) Maximum-intensity projection of aorta showing postsurgical situation at coarctation site (arrowhead). RV, right ventricle; LV, left ventricle

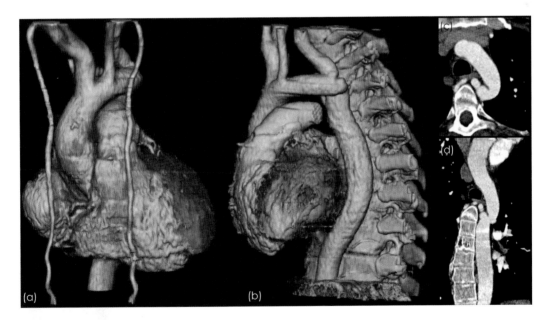

Figure 15.6 Coarctation of aorta. (a) and (b) Volume-rendered images of aorta from anterior and lateral views. (c) and (d) Multiplanar-reconstructed images of aorta with coarctation of the aorta

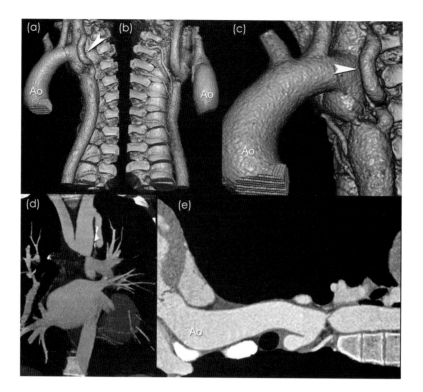

Figure 15.7 Coarctation of aorta. (a)–(c) Volume-rendered images of aorta with coarctation of the aorta. Bypass between left subclavian artery and thoracic aorta (arrowhead). (d) and (e) Maximum-intensity projection and curved multiplanar-reconstructed images of aorta showing clearly the coarctation with severe narrowing. Ao, aorta

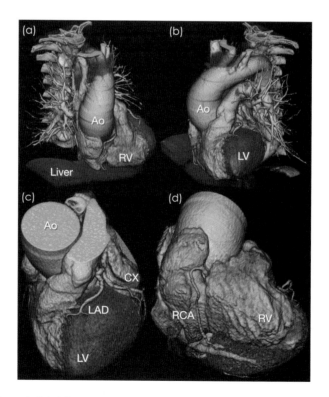

Figure 15.8 Dilatation of aortic root. (a)–(d) Volume-rendered images of heart and ascending aorta (Ao). The aortic root is dilated. LV, left ventricle; RV, right ventricle; LAD, left anterior descending; LCX, left circumflex; RCA, right coronary artery

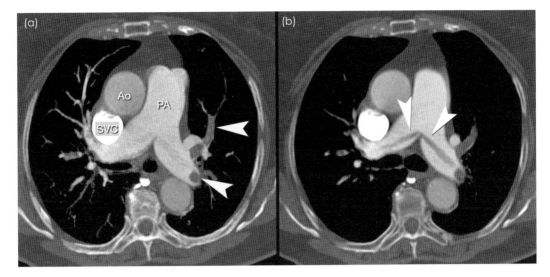

Figure 15.9 Pulmonary embolism. (a) Cross-sectional image of pulmonary artery (PA) and main branches. Filling defects in left pulmonary branch (lower arrowhead) and occluded smaller pulmonary branch (upper arrowhead). (b) Large filling defect at bifurcation of the main pulmonary artery (arrowheads). Ao, aorta; SVC, superior vena cava

REFERENCES

1. Nienaber CA, Eagle KA. Aortic dissection: new frontiers in diagnosis and management: Part I: from etiology to diagnostic strategies. Circulation 2003; 108: 628–35

2. Nienaber CA, Eagle KA. Aortic dissection: new frontiers in diagnosis and management: Part II: therapeutic management and follow-up. Circulation 2003; 108: 772–8

3. Nienaber CA, von Kodolitsch Y, Petersen B, et al. Intramural hemorrhage of the thoracic aorta. Diagnostic and therapeutic implications. Circulation 1995; 92: 1465–72

4. Coady MA, Rizzo JA, Hammond GL, et al. Penetrating ulcer of the thoracic aorta: what is it? How do we recognize it? How do we manage it? J Vasc Surg 1998; 27: 1006–15, discussion 1015–16

5. Drucker EA, Rivitz SM, Shepard JA, et al. Acute pulmonary embolism: assessment of helical CT for diagnosis. Radiology 1998; 209: 235–41

6. Rathbun SW, Raskob GE, Whitsett TL. Sensitivity and specificity of helical computed tomography in the diagnosis of pulmonary embolism: a systematic review. Ann Intern Med 2000; 132: 227–32

CHAPTER 16

Non-cardiac findings on cardiac computed tomography

Cardiac computed tomography not only provides information about the heart, great vessels and coronary arteries, but also includes a portion of the lungs, mediastinum, chest wall, spine and upper abdomen. Inevitably examinations of these additional structures will produce incidental findings that may be clinically insignificant, but which may also be of clinical importance such as early cancer (Figures 16.1–16.6). Expertise is required accurately to interpret both cardiac and non-cardiac incidental findings.

Two studies have reported the prevalence of significant non-cardiac findings on CT calcium screening examinations[1,2]. Horton et al. examined 1326 consecutive patients who were a mixture of asymptomatic self-referrals, asymptomatic individuals referred by their primary-care physician and symptomatic patients referred by either the primary-care physician or cardiologist[1]. There were 849 male and 477 female subjects with an average age of 55.4 years (range 23–87 years). Seventy-five per cent were non-smokers. Of these 1326

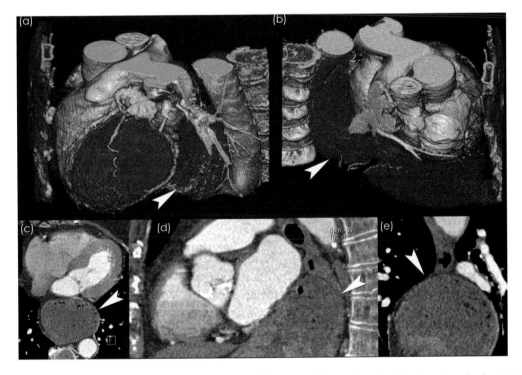

Figure 16.1 Large hiatal hernia. (a) and (b) Volume-rendered images of thorax showing the heart and a large mass in close proximity to the heart (arrowheads). (c) and (d) Multiplanar-reconstructed images revealed a mass posterior (c) to the heart contours (d) (arrowheads) compressing the left atrium. (e) Coronal reformatted plane of hernia (arrowhead)

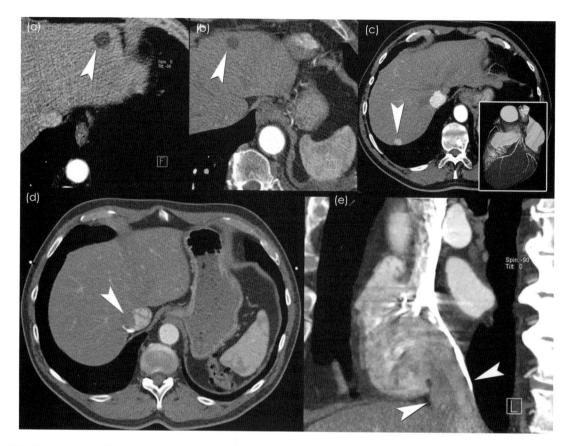

Figure 16.2 Liver abnormalities: (a) and (b) hypodense liver cysts (arrowheads); (c) hemangioma of liver; and (d) and (e) pseudothrombus of vena cava inferior due to non-homogeneous distribution of contrast material (arrowhead) and pseudo-obstruction of vena cava inferior (arrowheads e)

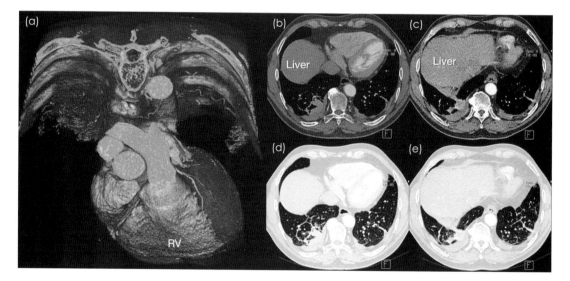

Figure 16.3 Lung atelectasis. (a) Volume-rendered image of heart, posterior thoracic cavity with spine and ribs. (b)–(e) Axial images showing heart and liver. The posterior pleura is thickened and posterior lower lobes of lung show areas of atelectasis on both sides. RV, right ventricle

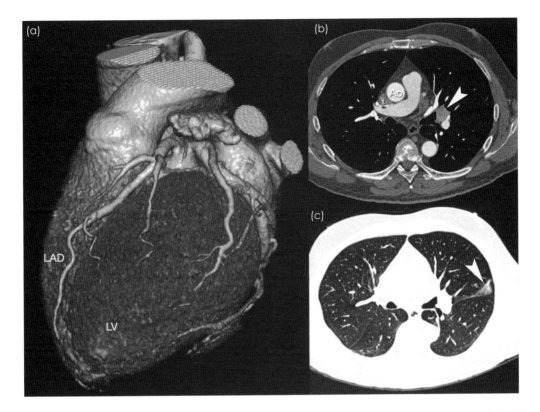

Figure 16.4 Lung carcinoma. (a) Volume-rendered image of the heart with normal left coronary arteries. (b) Axial image with tumor at left lung hilum (arrowhead). (c) Axial image with segmental lung atelectasis (arrowhead). LAD, left anterior descending; LV, left ventricle; Ao, aorta

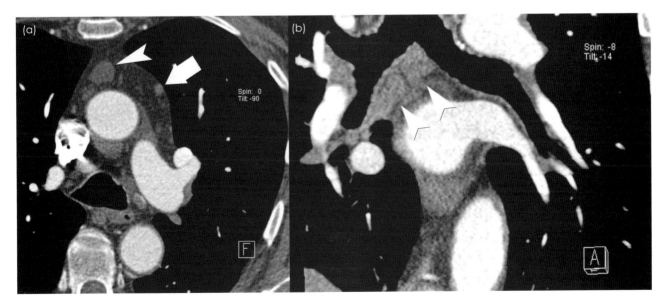

Figure 16.5 Lymph nodes in mediastinum. (a) and (b) Axial images demonstrating small lymph nodes (thick arrow) and large lymph node below the trachea carina (large arrowheads) in the anterior mediastinum

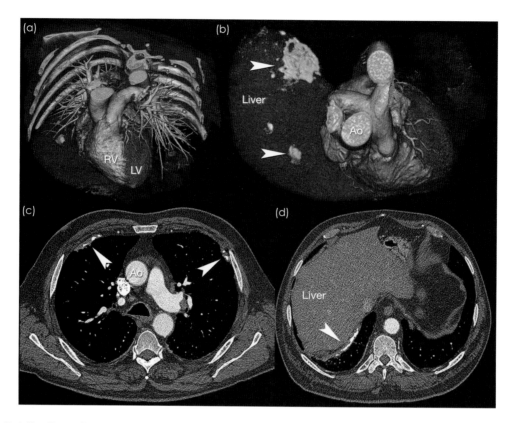

Figure 16.6 Calcifications of pleura. (a) and (b) Volume-rendered images of thorax. Large calcifications of the pleura at the right diaphragmatic site (arrowheads). (c) and (d) Calcifications of pleura at various localizations (arrowheads). RV, right ventricle; LV, left ventricle; Ao, aorta

patients, 103 (7.8%) had significant extracardiac pathology requiring additional work-up. The pathological abnormalities are listed in Table 16.1.

Hunold *et al.* reported on the prevalence of clinically significant incidental non-coronary findings in 1812 consecutive patients with known or suspected coronary artery disease who underwent electron-beam CT (EBCT) scanning for coronary artery calcification[2]. The mean age was 59 ± 16 years (range 20–86). Of the patients, 1407 (78%) were men and 405 (22%) were women. The investigators found a total of 2055 non-coronary pathological findings in 953 (53%) of the patients (Table 16.2). The most frequent findings were calcifications of various organs, in particular aortic calcium and heart valve calcification. The majority of these incidental findings were not considered to be of clinical relevance. Further diagnostic procedures were deemed to be necessary in 191 (11%) of the patients, 74% of which concerned the heart. In 22 (1.2%) of the patients specific treatment was instituted. Malignant disease was detected in three patients (0.2%) .

Table 16.1 Significant non-cardiac findings on CT coronary calcium examinations in 1326 patients[1]

	n
Non-calcified lung nodules < 1 cm	53
Lung nodules > 1 cm	12
Infiltrates	24
Indeterminate liver disease	7
Sclerotic bone lesions	2
Breast abnormalities	2
Polycystic liver disease	1
Esophageal thickening	1
Ascites	1
Total number with non-cardiac findings	103 (7.8%)

These two studies raise an extremely important question concerning the responsibility for interpretation of the cardiac CT scan. Who should read the scans: the cardiologist or the radiologist? The radiologist is specifically trained in the detection and interpretation of thoracic and abdominal scans, whereas the cardiologist is

Table 16.2 Incidence of non-coronary findings on EBCT coronary calcium screening in 1812 consecutive patients. A total of 2055 incidental findings were present in 953 (53%) of the patients[2]

	Incidental findings		Diagnostic consequences (n)	Therapeutic consequences (n)
	%	(n)		
Heart (pericardium, valves, cavities)	33	676	136	11
Aorta	28	564	9	6
Lung	28	564	13	3
Mediastinum	4	72	12	1
Abdominal organs	3	71	16	1
Spinal column	5	101	0	0

more specifically trained in the interpretation of the cardiovascular scan and much less so in other areas. It, therefore, seems that it is in the best interest of the patient that the examinations are interpreted in close cooperation between the cardiologist and the radiologist.

This issue may become even more important with the introduction of contrast-enhanced CT coronary angiography, which may become a widely used alternative investigation for diagnostic coronary angiography.

CONCLUSION

The incidence of significant non-coronary incidental findings on CT scan ranges between 7.8% and 11%, which may have diagnostic and subsequent treatment consequences. Correct identification and interpretation of incidental findings requires specific expertise which is probably best guaranteed by combined reading of the CT scans by a radiologist and cardiologist.

REFERENCES

1. Horton KM, Post WS, Blumenthal RS, Fishman EK. Prevalence of significant noncardiac findings on electron-beam computed tomography coronary artery calcium screening examinations. Circulation 2002; 106: 532–4

2. Hunold P, Schmermund A, Seibel RM, et al. Prevalence and clinical significance of accidental findings in electron-beam tomographic scans for coronary artery calcification. Eur Heart J 2001; 22: 1748–58

CHAPTER 17

Assessment of left ventricular function

CT scanning of the heart permits the evaluation of both the coronary arteries and left ventricular function, because three-dimensional data of the complete cardiac cycle are acquired during retrospectively gated multislice CT (MSCT) coronary angiography. To evaluate the coronary arteries, datasets are normally reconstructed during the mid-to-end diastolic phase to obtain (nearly) motion-free image quality. However, additional datasets can be reconstructed, e.g. every 5 or 10% of the cardiac cycle. Therefore, from the same data acquired during MSCT coronary angiography, information concerning left ventricular function can be extracted. After reconstruction of a number of datasets covering the entire cardiac cycle, short-axis images at different levels (e.g. apical, mid and basal) of the ventricle and at different time points can be reconstructed using dedicated software (Figure 17.1).

Left ventricle volumes can be measured after semi-automatic contouring of the ventricular cavity, and summation of the short-axis images applying Simpson's rule. These results can be plotted in a volume/time curve, allowing reliable identification of the end-systolic and end-diastolic phase and calculation of stroke volume, ejection fraction and (time-to) peak filling rate (Figure 17.2 and Table 17.1). After drawing additional epicardial contours of the left ventricle, quantitative information concerning left ventricular wall motion, thickening and thickness can be derived[3].

Recent studies demonstrated a good correlation of assessment of left ventricular volumes and ejection fraction between MSCT and MRI, biplane ventriculography[1,2] or echo cardiography[1–3]. The left ventricular ejection fraction determined by MSCT is reasonably accurate, but slight underestimation is noted because the end-systolic left ventricular volume is slightly overestimated owing to insufficient temporal resolution of

CT to determine the precise end-systolic time point. Grude et al. compared magnetic resonance determined global left ventricular myocardial function with four-slice MSCT data[2]. They found close agreement with

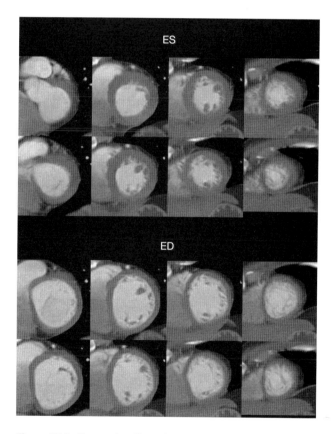

Figure 17.1 Reconstruction of short-axis images of the left ventricle obtained at the end-diastolic (ED) and end-systolic (ES) phase allows quantification (after semi-automatic contouring of the endocardial and epicardial border of the left ventricle) of stroke volume, ejection fraction and peak filling rate. This patient with a history of acute myocardial infarction had an impaired thickening of the apical part of the septum

end-diastolic volumes but less so with end-systolic volumes which resulted in an underestimation of left ventricular ejection fraction (Table 17.2).

Multislice CT is less reliable for the assessment of regional wall motion abnormalities when compared to established techniques such as biplane ventriculography, MRI or echocardiography. An early study performed with a four-row MSCT scanner found a close agreement between normal, akinetic and dyskinetic ventricular segments when compared with two-dimensional echocardiography, but only a moderate agreement in hypokinetic segments. Of the 79 segments with an abnormal wall motion on two-dimensional echocardiography, 68 were identified by CT[3]. Evaluation of the

Table 17.1 Left ventricular function parameters (see Figure 17.1)

Cardiac function		Normal range (M) (CT)
Ejection fraction (EF) (%)	55.0	56.00–78.00
End-diastolic volume (EDV) (ml)	228.6	77.00–195.00
End-systolic volume (ESV) (ml)	102.9	19.00–72.00
Stroke volume (SV) (ml)	125.6	51.00–133.00
Cardiac output (CO) (l/min)	5.90	2.82–8.82
Myocardial mass (at ED) (g)	124.1	118.00–238.00
Myocardial mass (avg) (g)	122.1±11.8	118.00–238.00

ED, end-diastole

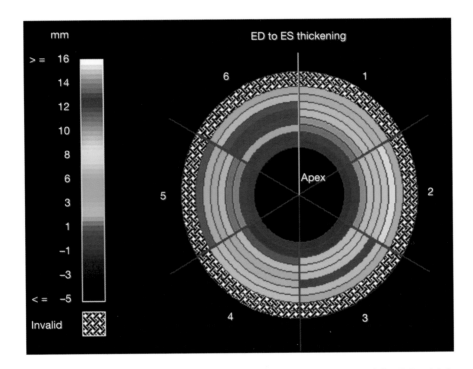

Figure 17.2 Bull's eye view of left ventricular wall thickening. (1)–(6) Anterior, anterolateral, inferolateral, inferoseptal, septal and anteroseptal sectors, respectively. ED, end-diastole; ES, end-systole

Table 17.2 Volumetric and functional left ventricular parameters[2]

	MSCT	Magnetic resonance imaging
Left ventricular end-diastolic volume (ml)	147±27	133±27
Left ventricular end-systolic volume (ml)	65±22	48±19
Left ventricular stroke volume (ml)	82±15	85±17
Left ventricular ejection fraction (%)	56±9	65±8

ventricular performance adds important functional information to the MSCT coronary angiographic examination. An advantage is the ability to scan the entire heart in a single breath hold (Figures 17.3 and 17.4).

However, one should be aware that in patients who undergo MSCT coronary angiography, beta-blocker are often administered prior to the examination. This may negatively affect the left ventricular performance. It is

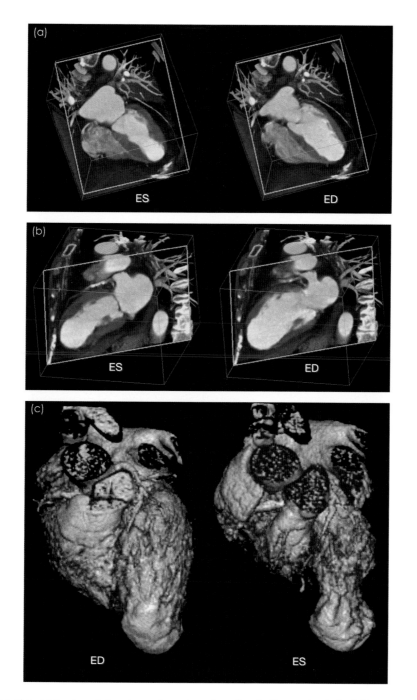

Figure 17.3 (a) Cross-section of the heart showing a four-chamber view in the end-systolic (ES) and end-diastolic (ED) phase, while the remaining volume remains visible. This patient had a previous myocardial infarction resulting in an aneurysm of the left ventricle. (b) Cross-section of the heart showing a two-chamber view in the end-systolic and end-diastolic phase of the same patient. (c) Volume-rendered images of the end-systolic and end-diastolic phase of the same patient. The presence of a left ventricular aneurysm is visualized, and the apex is not contracting

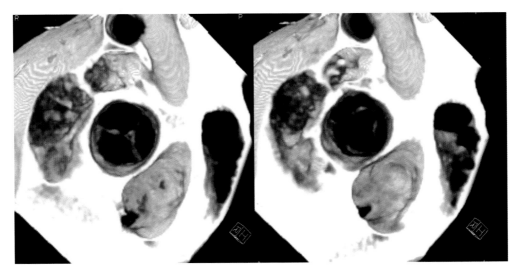

Figure 17.4 Reconstruction of the end-diastolic and end-systolic phase at the level of the aortic root shows the opening and closing of the aortic valve and allows assessment of valve function

of note that the assessment of left ventricular performance using MSCT can be a reliable alternative in patients with contraindications for MRI, considered to be the reference standard LV evaluation technique for instance in patients with pacemakers.

Crude evaluation of cardiac valve function is also possible (Figure 17.4).

CONCLUSION

CT allows comprehensive cardiac examination including assessment of the coronary arteries and the left ventricular function.

REFERENCES

1.   Juergens KU, Grude M, Fallenberg EM, et al. Using ECG-gated multidetector CT to evaluate global left ventricular myocardial function in patients with coronary artery disease. Am J Roentgenol 2002; 179: 1545–50

2.   Grude M, Juergens KU, Wichter T, et al. Evaluation of global left ventricular myocardial function with electrocardiogram-gated multidetector computed tomography: comparison with magnetic resonance imaging. Invest Radiol 2003; 38: 653–61

3.   Dirksen MS, Bax JJ, de Roos A, et al. Usefulness of dynamic multislice computed tomography of left ventricular function in unstable angina pectoris and comparison with echocardiography. Am J Cardiol 2002; 90: 1157–60

CHAPTER 18

Artifacts

An artifact is defined as a distortion or error in an image that is not related to the structure being imaged[1]. Artifacts can be divided into two main categories:

(1) Artifacts that are inherent to the technical design of the scanner or inherent to the physics of the technique. For instance, using black and white film creates black and white images. This generates an artifact because the color is missing owing to the technical limitation of film that can only create black and white images.

(2) Artifacts that are generated in the application of the technique. For instance, the shutter speed of a camera falls short if the object to be photographed moves faster than the shutter speed, which results in a blurred image.

Artifacts may also be defined as an inaccurate representation of the structure being imaged. The degree of inaccuracy may be small and have no impact on the diagnostic information of the image or may be large and severely distort the diagnostic information.

Coronary imaging is considered to be the ultimate challenge to CT because the coronary arteries are small, tortuous and subject to significant motion owing to cardiac contraction and inspiration[2,3]. This places optimal demands on the technique in terms of temporal, spatial and contrast resolution, that cannot always be met. For instance, the speed of motion during systole is too fast for the specifications of the CT scanner. Thus, to achieve optimal 'artifact-free' coronary images the acquisition should be fast (short temporal resolution), the voxels should be small (high x-y-z axis resolution) and the attenuation value should be high (optimal contrast resolution)[4].

Adequate knowledge about artifacts is necessary to prevent their generation, or if they occur should help identification and interpretation.

TEMPORAL RESOLUTION

Temporal resolution is of paramount importance in the imaging of moving organs (Figure 18.1). An object can move at a certain speed and a sharp image of the object can be obtained only if the time required to obtain the image is faster than the speed, of motion of the object. In cardiac CT, temporal resolution is the time required for the acquisition of data that are used to generate one image.

Temporal resolution in CT imaging depends mainly on the gantry rotation time and the image reconstruction algorithm. The algorithms for image reconstruction are defined based on the number of segments that they can use to reconstruct one image. The 180° of gantry rotation that are required to generate one image can be obtained from the same cardiac cycle (e.g. single segment) or from more than one consecutive cardiac cycle (e.g. multisegment). In principle, a single-segment algorithm should be preferred at low heart rates (< 70 bpm) and whenever possible. For high heart rates (> 70 bpm), multisegment algorithms may improve image quality.

It is obvious that the slower the motion of the object the better the images. Therefore, using a fixed temporal window, the balance between the speed of acquisition and the speed of the object can be improved by slowing down the motion of the object. This is the reason why several centers suggest using negative chronotropic drugs prior to the scan to reduce the heart rate. Respiratory or other voluntary or non-voluntary motion

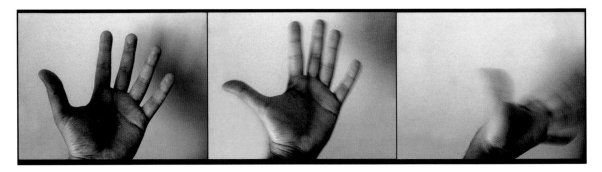

Aquisition speed
> object speed

Aquisition speed
~ object speed

Aquisition speed
< object speed

Figure 18.1 Temporal resolution. The relationship between speed of image acquisition and speed of motion of the object to be imaged determines the amount of blurring that will be displayed. Ideally, the speed of image acquisition should be much faster than the speed of the object. In cardiac CT these two factors depend equally on the heart rate and the reconstruction algorithm

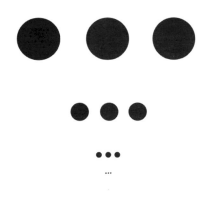

Figure 18.2 Spatial resolution. The capability of a technique to separate two neighboring objects defines its spatial resolution

artifacts can only be reduced by other measures, including breath hold and lying still on the couch.

SPATIAL RESOLUTION

Spatial resolution is the capability to discern two small objects (Figure 18.2). It depends on several different parameters related to the CT scanner. Most of the parameters that affect spatial resolution cannot be modified by the operator (focal spot size, detector size, distance between focal spot and detector ring, number of projections, etc.). The operator instead can modify other parameters in the scan and reconstruction phases (e.g. collimation, reconstruction increment, field of view, fil-

tering, etc.) to exploit the maximal spatial resolution allowed by the CT scanner.

CONTRAST RESOLUTION

The degree of contrast to differentiate between tissues with varying attenuation characteristics is defined as contrast resolution (Figure 18.3). Because CT has a much better contrast resolution than conventional radiography, tissues with only very small differences in density can be distinguished. The contrast resolution is affected by a number of fixed factors such as the detector sensitivity and patient size. Factors that can be influenced include the radiation intensity (the X-ray tube's current and voltage), slice thickness, reconstruction filtering and image noise. Additionally, the display of the tissue contrast is affected by the window settings. The display size and the distance between the observer and the screen influence the perception of contrast resolution. Image noise, which is the fluctuation of the measurement compared to the nominal density, affects contrast resolution. The amount of noise is related to a number of the factors mentioned above, including the radiation intensity, slice thickness and detector size.

NOISE

Noise can be exemplified as the 'fog' when looking out of the window. Depending on the amount and density of the water particles in the air the image that is seen

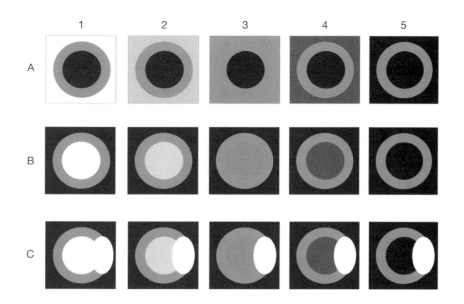

Figure 18.3 Contrast resolution. Contrast resolution defines the capability of a technique to discriminate between objects when their imaging properties are similar. In the first example (row A, 1–5) a round object with a black core surrounded by a gray ring is set into a background that varies from white (1) to black (5). In the middle panel (3), the background is similar to the ring of the object so that it disappears, while the black core remains visible. In the second example (row B, 1–5) a rounded object with a white core and a gray ring is set into a black background. The color of the core varies from white (1) to black (5). This causes the core of the object to merge with the surrounding ring when their colors become similar. In the third example (row C, 1–5) the same object as in row B is displayed, that in this case can be regarded as a cross-sectional view of a coronary vessel. The background is black because it is fat tissue, the ring around the object is gray like the vessel wall (i.e. endothelium, tunica media, adventitia and eventually plaque tissue) and the core of the object (i.e. vessel lumen) is a variable color depending on the vascular enhancement. In addition, a white object (i.e. calcification in the vessel wall) is added to the gray ring. The variation of the color of the lumen from white (1) to black (5) shows how the respective components of the coronary artery are visualized. In particular, too high an enhancement in the lumen prevents adequate depiction of the borders of the calcification in the vessel wall (1), while the absence of enhancement prevents the visualization of the lumen (3). The ideal situation occurs when the vessel enhancement has a value that is in between that of the calcification and the vessel wall. The cases represented in (4) and (5) are of no clinical use because they presuppose the presence of a negative contrast within the vessel lumen

becomes progressively fuzzy and contours are more difficult to detect.

The noise in the CT image is the variability of the attenuation value between two neighboring voxels compared to the average attenuation measured in that area (Figure 18.4). Ideally, a perfect scanner would produce images with extremely low noise so that when the operator measures the attenuation in the vessel lumen the resulting value would be almost the same in neighboring voxels. Commercially available scanners can produce images with very low noise but at the 'price' of a high dose of radiation. One of the main factors that determine the noise in the image is the number of milliamperes per second produced by the X-ray tube. Increasing the milliamperes per second will increase the number of photons that can hit the detector, thereby increasing the ratio between signal and noise.

Another factor affecting image noise is the absorption of the patient. In patients with normal weight and length, the X-ray dose should be adjusted depending on the specific scanner. Preset protocols and experience usually enable the correct dose to be identified. A low X-ray dose is desirable; however, it reduces image quality. When the ratio between the X-ray dose and the patient's absorption is too low the scan can be too noisy and therefore not assessable (Figure 18.5).

There are two situations in which the radiation dose must be increased. The *first* is in large patients with a significant amount of soft tissue surrounding the thorax (Figure 18.6). More soft tissue means that the radiation is absorbed and fewer photons strike the detector array, which results in increased noise. The *second* is in women with large breasts (Figure 18.7). Here the presence of a large amount of fat tissue absorbs photons again causing increased noise. In both cases, a physical examination

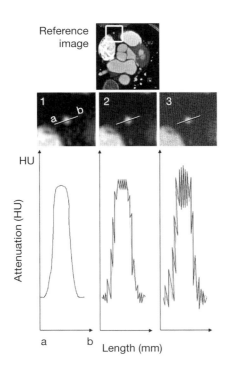

Figure 18.4 Graphic representation of image noise. The box represents a region of interest from the reference axial image obtained at the mid-segment of the right coronary artery. In (1)–(3) noise is progressively added. The attenuation values along the line a–b are then plotted in the length–attenuation graphs. The first example (1) shows the case of very low noise and the corresponding graph displays a smooth curve in the transition between a and b. In examples (2) and (3), the increase in noise causes a progressively larger oscillation of the attenuation values. This example explains why images with noise are more difficult to evaluate

and/or scans that precede the coronary CT angiography would identify the situation and a higher X-ray dose should be given.

Definite values of milliamperes cannot be provided because they depend on the specific characteristics of each specific scanner (e.g. rotation time, X-ray tube power, etc.). As a guideline, once the operator has defined a protocol that provides an optimal image quality in 'standard patients', the milliamperes should be increased by 15–20% in large-sized patients or women with large breasts. In cases of extremely large patients or breasts, the number of milliamperes should be set to the maximum allowed by the scanner.

When noise increases in the images (Figure 18.8), the capability to discern objects is impaired regardless of the spatial resolution and can result in non-diagnostic image quality and therefore scan failure.

PARTIAL VOLUME, INTERPOLATION AND FILTERING

Partial volume (also known as 'volume averaging') is an artifact that occurs in all voxels of all images when differences in attenuation are present between neighboring structures. It depends on the fact that voxels are much larger than the structures that they represent. For instance, in a voxel of $0.3 \times 0.3 \times 0.3$ mm, a submillimetric structure such as endothelium cannot be represented (Figure 18.9). Therefore, it will be averaged with other surrounding structures such as the vessel lumen and inner layers of the vessel wall (i.e. adventitia). The final appearance of the voxel where the endothelium lies will be the result of the averaged attenuation of all the structures that are present.

Interpolation averages the attenuation across neighboring and distant pixels/voxels. It is used to create data and fill the gap between two known points. This becomes particularly evident in areas of the image where there is a very large attenuation gradient. Examples of these areas are the edge between air and soft tissues in the lung parenchyma, and the edge between calcium and soft tissue in the coronary artery walls.

Partial volume and interpolation cause so-called 'blooming' as can be seen with calcium, contrast material and surgical clips in the coronary arteries. These highly attenuating structures appear to be much larger than their actual size because of the averaging within the voxel and interpolation between all the neighboring voxels (Figure 18.10).

Filtering reduces this effect. Filters are designed to enhance the edges between structures with different attenuations. This procedure tries to restore the balance between the need for adequate interpolation (that smooths the image) and the need for adequate detection of edges (that sharpens the image). Unfortunately, filtering increases the noise of the image; therefore, the operator should identify the correct balance between filtering and noise to obtain sharper images.

BEAM-HARDENING ARTIFACTS

Beam-hardening artifacts occur when the radiation is completely absorbed by an object with extremely high attenuation (Table 18.1). The effect can be compared to a shield for the X-ray beam. The human body modifies the photon spectrum of the heterochromic X-ray beam.

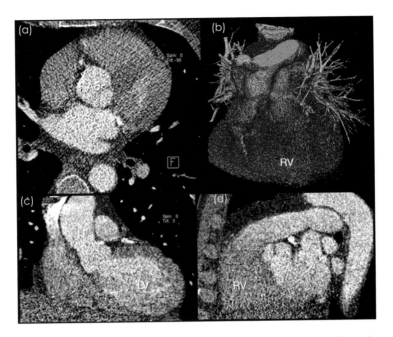

Figure 18.5 Noise causing scan failure. The cardiac CT scan result may be too noisy when the ratio between the X-ray attenuation by the patient and the X-ray dose is too high. The images reconstructed from a dataset with excessive noise cannot be improved. The noise in the axial image (a) does not allow adequate images to be achieved with volume rendering (b), or with coronal (c) or sagittal (d) multiplanar views. Ao, aorta; LV, left ventricle; RV, right ventricle

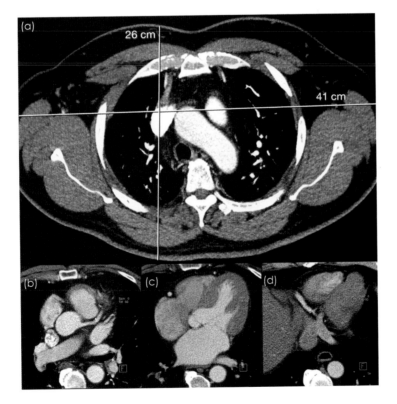

Figure 18.6 Coronary CT of a large patient. In patients with a high body weight or body mass, the scan power has to be set to a maximum to produce images of diagnostic quality. In this example a patient weighting > 100 kg was scanned with a tube load of 725 mA/s and a rotation time of 375 ms (a). The generated axial images at different levels (b)–(d) are of diagnostic image quality

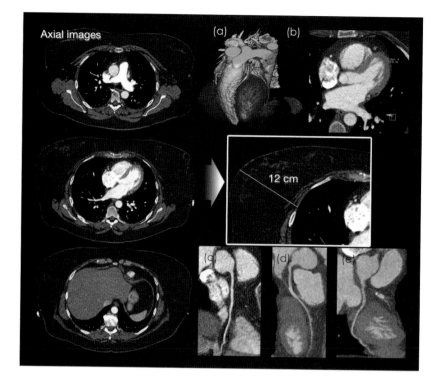

Figure 18.7 Cardiac CT of woman with large breasts. The ratio between patient's X-ray absorption and X-ray dose should be optimized in the presence of a large breast. In this example a patient was scanned with a tube load of 720 mA/s and a rotation time of 375 ms. The panoramic axial images in the left panel show the amount of tissue that surrounds the thorax (see thickness in the white box). The three-dimensional volume rendering (a) and axial images (b) are of sufficient image quality. The curved multiplanar reconstruction of the right coronary artery (c), left anterior descending (d) and left circumflex, although noisy, are also of diagnostic image quality

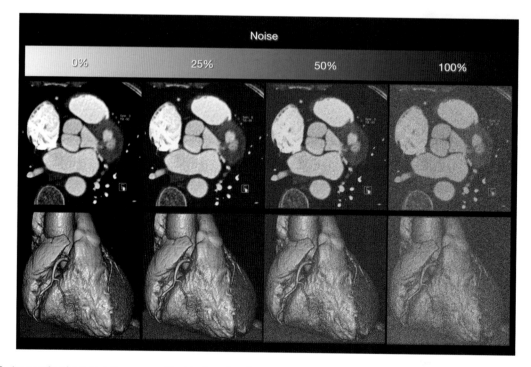

Figure 18.8 Increasing image noise exemplified in the visualization of the right coronary artery

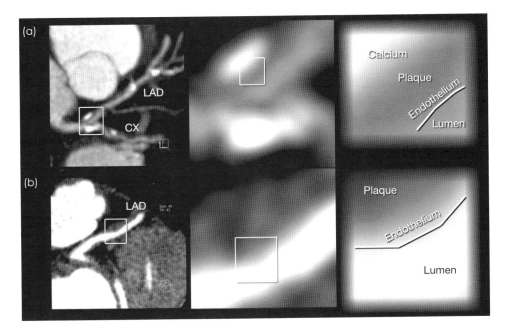

Figure 18.9 Volume averaging. Volume averaging is an artifact that affects all images in the dataset. (a) Mixed plaque (calcific and non-calcific plaque) in the left anterior descending artery (LAD). The progressive magnification of the plaque in the transition area between calcium, plaque and lumen displays how the microscopic structures such as endothelium cannot be distinguished. This is also the case in a non-calcific plaque (b). CX, circumflex artery

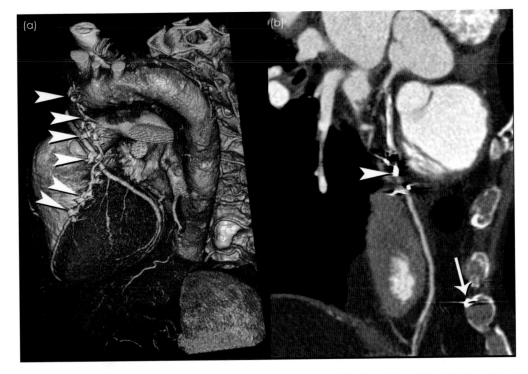

Figure 18.10 Volume averaging from surgical clips. Surgical clips used to close the branches of the left internal mammary artery are clearly displayed in the three-dimensional volume-rendering image (a). They appear to be much larger than their actual size because of the volume-averaging effect (arrowheads). In a curved-multiplanar reconstruction (b) showing the left anterior descending artery the presence of the surgical clips causes artifacts at the anastomoses between the vessel and the left internal mammary artery (arrowhead). The wires used to fix the sternum after sternotomy generate the same type of artifact (arrow)

Table 18.1 Type, cause and management of artifacts

Type	Problem	Cause	Solution	Practical advice
Motion	high heart rate	insufficient temporal resolution	scan heart rate < 70 bpm for visualization of the entire coronary tree	at heart rate >70bpm the scan can be performed but complete visualization of the coronary tree will not be possible. If the indication of the scan is proximal coronary obstructive disease, scan with heart rate <90bpm can be performed even though with a lower rate of success when compared to a lower heart rate
	irregular heart rate	atrial fibrillation other irregularities insufficient temporal resolution	scan regular heart rate medication ECG editing abort	for irregularities characterized by a defined QRS complex and at least intermittent diastolic periods >500 ms it is still possible to perform ECG editing
		too short diastolic phase	ECG editing	before the scan evaluate the presence of extrasystole. When extrasystole present on a sinus rhythm <65 bpm the ECG editing is always feasible
		extrasystole triggered during breath hold	test the apnea prior to the scan and look for extrasystole	test apnea prior to the scan
	patient breathing	poor patient instructions	thoroughly instruct the patient	
		stressed patient	perform more than one test for apnea	
		language barrier	adapt language	the referring physician should properly address this type of patient
		partial or total deafness	trigger breath hold with a visual signal (if available on the scanner)	ensure the technician talks to the patient prior to the scan
	breath hold control	Valsalva maneuver	instruct and test the patient to prevent Valsalva maneuver	Valsalva maneuver impairs the ability to remain still and also prevents the inflow of contrast material from the subclavian vein because of the increased intra thoracic pressure
		too deep inspiratory breath hold	instruct and test the patient's ability to perform a normal inspiratory breath hold	too deep an inspiratory breath hold impairs the ability to remain still

Continued.

Table 18.1 continued

Type	Problem	Cause	Solution	Practical advice
	patient voluntary motion	hot sensation from contrast material	warn the patient about the heat he/she will experience during the scan	
		coughing/sneezing	warn the patient about the importance of staying still during the breath hold and eventually use medication to reduce the symptoms	
	patient involuntary motion	diaphragmatic drift	reduce scan time	with a scan time of 15–20 s a certain amount of diaphragmatic drift cannot be avoided; with a scan time of < 10 s the impact of diaphragmatic drift will be significantly reduced
Image contrast/ noise	blurry and fuzzy	inadequate ratio between X-ray dose and patient's absorption		the overwhelming noise in the image can prevent adequate diagnostic evaluation of coronary arteries; for patients > 100 kg use the maximum dose allowed by the scanner compatible with patient's age
	images 'large' patient	high tissue absorption throughout the dataset;	increase mA/s	
	'very large' breast	high tissue absorption in the distal part of the dataset	increase mA/s	the overwhelming noise in the image can prevent adequate diagnostic evaluation of the distal part of the coronary arteries; use the maximum dose allowed by the scanner compatible with patient's age
Beam hardening	streak artifacts	contrast material (SVC and right heart)	use bolus chaser	use the most 'diagnostic' radiation dose; a low dose of radiation is still too high if the diagnosis cannot be made
		pacemaker wires, prosthetic valves, surgical clips, indicators at the anastomosis site of bypass grafts, sternal wires, calcium, stents, clips	increase mA/s	
				use higher convolution filters
Volume averaging	'blooming'	contrast material	use bolus chaser	use the most 'diagnostic' radiation dose; a low dose of radiation is still too high if the diagnosis cannot be made
		calcium, stents, clips	increase mA/s	use higher convolution filters

Continued.

Table 18.1 continued

Type	Problem	Cause	Solution	Practical advice
Temporal window	misregistration of data in one isolated stack of images	patient motion	improve patient instructions	
	motion in segment 2 (mid-RCA)	suboptimal selection of temporal window	try a different reconstruction window (±50 ms/±10%)	think ahead: optimization should be 'per vessel' rather than per data set
	diffuse but not large motion especially on the RCA	suboptimal selection of temporal window	try a different reconstruction window (±50 ms/±10%)	
	large motion artifact in one isolated stack of images	extrasystole/premature heartbeat	exclude extrasystole with ECG editing	
	large motion artifact in multiple stacks of images	irregular ECG wave or irregular heart rhythm	check ECG automatic triggering and edit if necessary	
Missing data	lack of information at a defined level of the scan range	irregular ECG baseline	ECG editing	
		mistriggering	ECG editing	
		extra low heart rate (<40 bpm)	ECG editing	
		extrasystole with borderline heart rate	ECG editing	
	missed LM	scan start too low patient apnea during topogram was different from that during the angiography scan	re-scan the small proximal range after administering a 60-ml bolus of contrast material	perform dummy apnea
	missed PDA	scan ends too high patient apnea during topogram was different from that during the angiography scan	re-scan the small distal range after administering a 60-ml bolus of contrast material	use a scan range longer than required and end the scan manually when the real time images show the PDA

Continued.

Table 18.1 *continued*

Type	Problem	Cause	Solution	Practical advice
Vessel enhance-ment	poor enhancement	extremely fast circulation time (young patients, congenital anomalies of the great vessels of the thorax and heart)	start the scan visually and increase injection parameters (volume/rate/iodine)	
		early-triggering bolus tracking	streak artifacts from the SVC and projecting into the ROI, trigger the scan	position carefully the ROI in the middle of the ascending aorta and select a monitoring level not too close to the heart
		late-triggering bolus tracking	start the scan visually when the contrast material appears in the ascending aorta	
		low contrast injection rate	use > 3 ml/s	
		low contrast iodine	use > 350 mg/ml	
		low contrast volume	use no less than 10 ml	
		wrist IV	use antecubital access	
		partial extravasation of contrast	use large veins test veins with saline	
	no enhancement	injector not connected	connect injector	
		injector-tube disconnection	tighten injector-tube connection	
		extravasation	use large veins	
Image quality	noisy images	too low mAs	reduce filtering (will decrease confidence in stenosis evaluation)	
		'large' patient/breast	reduce filtering (will decrease confidence in stenosis evaluation)	
		evident noise but not in entire dataset	presence of premature heartbeats and prospective tube current modulation switched on	

ECG, electrocardiogram; LM, left main coronary artery; IV, intravenous; PDA, posterior descending artery; RCA, right coronary artery; ROI, region of interest; SVC, superior vena cava

High-energy photons are absorbed to a lesser extent, while low-energy photons are highly absorbed. Therefore, the average energy level of absorbed photons is shifted to the higher energies, that strike the detector array. This phenomenon causes beam-hardening artifacts. The significance of an artifact increases progressively with the degree of attenuation until it creates a shadow of attenuation on the opposite side of the object.

In cardiac imaging different objects have a high X-ray absorption: pacemaker wires, prosthetic valves, surgical clips, indicators at the anastomosis site of bypass grafts, sternal wires and stents. The pooling of high concentrations of contrast material in the superior vena cava and right atrium and ventricle can also cause beam-hardening artifacts.

Beam-hardening artifacts are annoying because they prevent adequate visualization of the surrounding structures (Figures 18.11 and 18.12). Unfortunately, to date, there is no good solution to avoid or handle this type of artifact.

MOTION ARTIFACTS

Motion artifacts are caused by motion of the patient or one of his/her parts in a non-expected or exaggerated manner (Table 18.1). A typical example of the former is respiratory motion when the patient is not supposed to breathe (Figure 18.13). A typical example of the latter is the motion of the coronary artery because of an inadequate ratio between the acquisition speed (e.g. temporal resolution) and the speed of the vessel (Figure 18.14).

The correct approach to motion artifacts starts before the scan. Most of the sources of motion artifacts can be managed properly with thorough patient selection and preparation. High heart rates (above 70 bpm) should be avoided (Figure 18.15); although it may be possible to achieve sufficient image quality with a high heart rate, the success rate is lower and parts of the coronary tree cannot be visualized.

Irregular heart rates are not an absolute contraindication to coronary CT angiography. While irregular heart rates characterized by a high ventricular response (> 70 bpm) amplify the problems described for high heart rates, mild heart rhythm irregularities with an average heart rate < 70 bpm can be managed in most cases (if the software allows ECG editing) during the reconstruction of the images (see below).

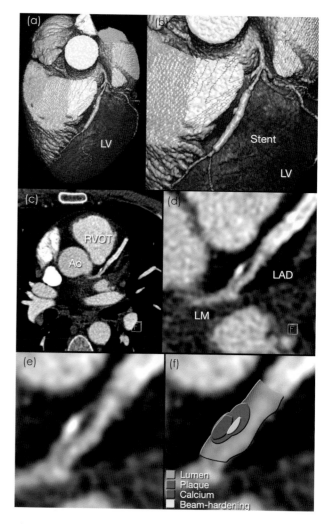

Figure 18.11 Beam hardening from coronary stents and calcium. A patient with a stent in the left anterior descending (LAD) is displayed with three-dimensional volume rendering (a) and (b). On the original axial images at the level of the proximal left anterior descending (c) and especially after magnification (d) a plaque can be visualized with both calcific and non-calcific parts. After further magnification (e) and labeling (f) several different components of the plaque can be identified. In particular, it is possible to see the dark region (yellow color in (f)) close to the calcific region (blue in (f)) of the plaque and projecting towards the lumen of the vessel (green in (f)). This region is not an actual low-attenuation region due to the presence of lipid material but it is a shadow due to beam-hardening artifact. Ao, ascending aorta; LM, left main coronary artery; LV, left ventricle; RV, right ventricle

Extrasystoles can be considered as mild heart rhythm irregularities, and are not a contraindication for coronary CT angiography unless they are very frequent (more than one in two heartbeats). It is wise to look for the occurrence or disappearance of extrasystoles during

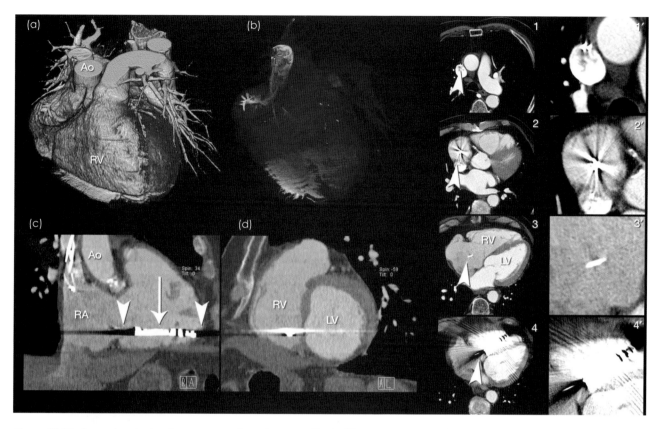

Figure 18.12 Beam hardening from pacemaker wires. A patient with a pacemaker is displayed with three-dimensional volume rendering with solid settings (a) and transparent settings (b). In the coronal (c) and sagittal (d) multiplanar planes the pacemaker wire (arrow) and beam-hardening artifacts (arrowheads) in the right heart are clearly displayed. In the right panel of the figure, axial images in a craniocaudal direction (1–4) are displayed and the position of the pacemaker wire is indicated (arrowheads). The magnification of the same images in the region of the pacemaker (1'–4') shows how large the artifacts can become depending on the orientation of the wire compared to that of the X-ray beams. In addition, volume averaging effects also play a role. The appearance of the pacemaker wire is much larger than the actual size due to this artifact. Ao, ascending aorta; RA, right atrium; LV, left ventricle; RV, right ventricle

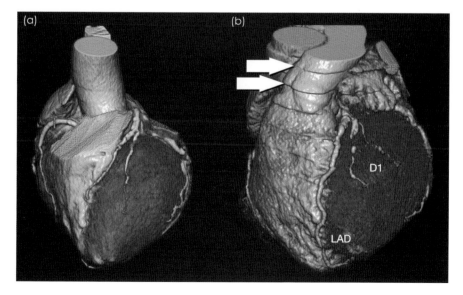

Figure 18.13 Voluntary motion. Two examples are displayed with three-dimensional volume rendering. (a) No voluntary motion is present. (b) Voluntary motion is present (arrows). LAD, left anterior descending; D1, first diagonal branch

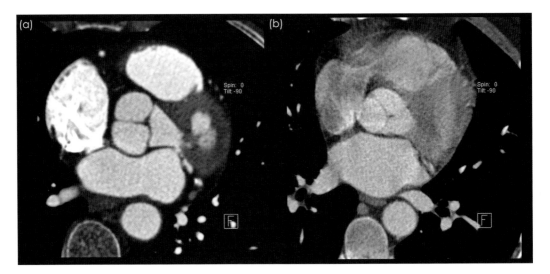

Figure 18.14 Involuntary motion. Two example axial images are displayed. (a) No motion is present and the structures of the heart are sharp. (b) Motion from heartbeat is present and all the relevant structures of the heart are blurred

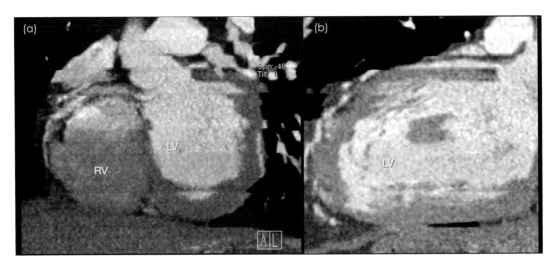

Figure 18.15 Motion artifacts resulting from high heart rate. High heart rates may cause deterioration of image quality. (a) Short-axis view of the right coronary artery. (b) Long axis view from the left anterior descending artery. The images were obtained from a patient with a heart rate of 120 bpm. LV, left ventricle; RV, right ventricle

breath holding prior to scan. This can be tested with a trial 15-s breath hold.

Patient breathing during the scan can cause scan failure (Figure 18.16). Therefore, the patient should be thoroughly instructed and tested in his/her breath holding prior to the scan. The operator should check that the patient performs an inspiratory breath hold without performing a Valsalva maneuver. The higher pressure generated during this maneuver can reduce the inflow of contrast material through the subclavian vein and the pressure can also impair the ability of the patient to stay still. Patients can also have difficulties in maintaining a still position when the breathhold is too deep (Figure 18.17). Nonetheless, with a required apnea of about 15–18 s, a deeper breath hold will provide a significant advantage. When the required apnea is longer the patient should be trained accordingly. It is then recommended that the patient be taught to perform an inspiratory breath hold without Valsalva maneuver.

In some cases the patient can move voluntarily during the scan because of the sudden heat sensation that rushes through the whole body (due to the intravenous administration of contrast material), which may cause coughing or sneezing. The operator should explain to

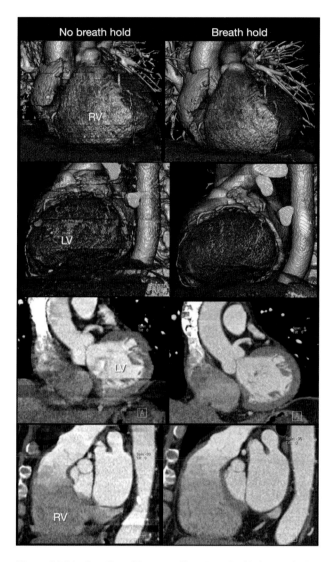

Figure 18.16 Cardiac CT scan without and with breathhold. The images obtained during a non-breath hold acquisition (left panels) cannot be evaluated. The only solution is to repeat the scan as displayed in the right panels. LV, left ventricle; RV, right ventricle

the patient the type of feeling he/she will experience to prevent coughing or sneezing.

Another source of non-voluntary motion, different from that determined by heart contraction, is the 'diaphragmatic drift'. This phenomenon occurs 8–10 s after the initiation of a standard breath hold. It consists of a slow and progressive motion of the diaphragm in the caudocranial direction. Usually, because it is slow and progressive, and it runs in one direction, it does not significantly affect the diagnostic quality of the images. It only enhances the misregistration between consecu-

tive stacks of images, creating steps. There is no means to avoid it; however, a shorter scan time (< 10 s) will probably significantly reduce the occurrence of diaphragmatic drift.

TEMPORAL WINDOW

The correct positioning of the temporal window within the cardiac cycle to obtain motion-free images is mandatory for a dataset of good quality. Unfortunately, there are few rules to identify the position within the diastolic phase where the motion of all coronary segments is minimized. Often, especially when the heart rate is not stable or with high heart rates, it is not possible to identify one single data set in which all segments are motion-free (Table 18.1).

The basic approach can be summarized as follows. After the end of the scan procedure the operator should perform a reconstruction in the mid-to-end diastolic phase starting at –400 ms before the R wave or at 60% of the R-to-R interval. When the images are not optimal in this dataset there two possibilities: the dataset is of good quality but one or more segments still have residual motion, or the dataset is not of diagnostic quality and there is residual motion along the entire coronary tree. In the first case, the operator should perform additional reconstruction with similar settings (e.g. –350/–450 ms or 55/65%). In the second case, the operator should perform a multiphasic reconstruction (i.e. 10–20 reconstructions at each 5–10% of the R-to-R interval) throughout the cardiac cycle to sample the best position for the temporal window.

In some cases the image quality of the dataset is good even though one single stack of images is misregistered (Figure 18.18). A small amount of misregistration can often be observed (Figure 18.19). In these cases no further datasets are required.

When residual motion is confined to the mid-right coronary artery a further dataset should be reconstructed with slightly earlier and slightly delayed temporal window settings.

When residual motion affects the entire right coronary artery a reconstruction should be performed at around 30% of the R-to-R interval.

When a stack of images looks completely out of registration while in the others no major motion artifact has been observed, the operator should inspect the ECG for the presence of premature beats (Figure 18.20).

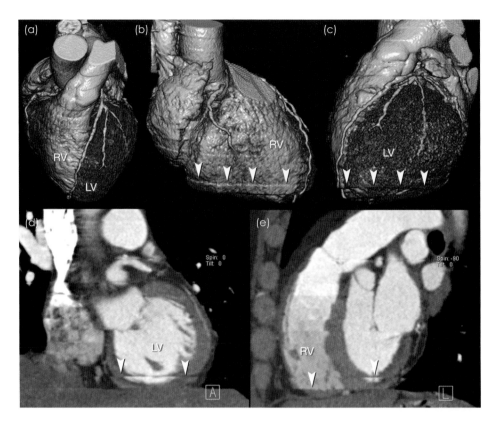

Figure 18.17 Respiratory-motion artifacts. In some cases the patient cannot perform a steady breath hold during the scan. At the end of the scan some motion artifacts may be observed. Volume rendering of the proximal part of the dataset shows a very good image quality (a). In the distal part of the dataset, there is misregistration between the stacks of images (arrowheads in (b) and (c)). Also, in the coronal (d) and sagittal (e) multiplanar views the presence of misregistration (arrowheads) can be appreciated. L, left ventricle; RV, right ventricle

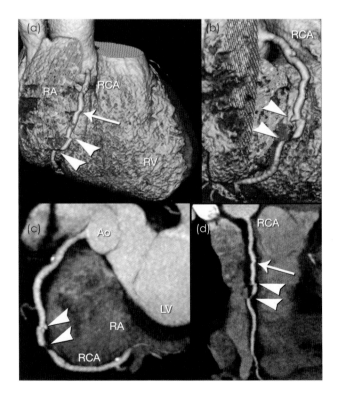

Figure 18.18 Severe misregistration artifact. In some cases, although the heart rate is optimal and there are no evident irregularities, one or more stacks of images can be misregistered. (a) Three-dimensional volume rendering displaying the right coronary artery (RCA). A high (arrowheads) and a lower (arrow) degree of misregistration are displayed. In the magnification of the image (b), the misregistration clearly causes an interruption in the continuity of the right coronary artery (arrowheads). Using maximum-intensity projection (c) in a plane parallel to the atrio-ventricular groove the configuration of the vessel also appears to be altered (arrowheads). In the curved multiplanar reconstruction (d) the appearance of the two sites of misregistration (arrowheads and arrow) is displayed. Ao, ascending aorta; RA, right atrium; LV, left ventricle; RV, right ventricle

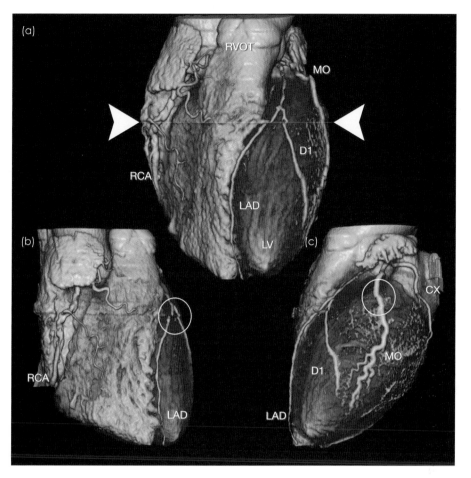

Figure 18.19 Subtle misregistration artifact. In some cases misregistration artifacts may be subtle. (a) Left anterior view using three-dimensional volume rendering. The location of the misregistration artifact is highlighted by the arrowheads and the horizontal line. The impact of this artifact on the integrity of the left anterior descending (LAD) (b) (white circle) and on the large marginal branch (MO) of the left circumflex (CX) (c) (white circle) is displayed. This artifact should not be mistaken for a stenosis. D1, first diagonal branch; RCA, right coronary artery; LV, left ventricle; RVOT, right ventricle outflow tract

MISSING DATA

When the ECG signal is low and noisy, the automatic triggering software can have problems in correctly detecting the R wave (Table 18.1). Therefore, the quality of the ECG signal and proper ECG triggering should always be checked by the operator before starting the reconstructions.

At high heart rates (> 70 bpm) some residual motion can often be observed. In these cases a multisegment reconstruction algorithm should be applied to reduce the effective temporal resolution. These algorithms differ slightly between manufacturers but are all based on the reconstruction of one image from two or more heart cycles. The use of these algorithms can improve image quality; however, the improvement is not always sufficient (Figures 18.21 and 18.22).

Data can be missed when the scan range is inadequately set. The main reasons for missing data are related to too short a scan range or to a discrepancy of the depth of patient's breath hold between the topogram and the angiographic scan.

The worst case occurs when the cranial part of the scan is missing, making it impossible to evaluate the left main coronary artery and the proximal branches. Missing data can also occur when the scan range ends too early and part of the posterior descending artery is missing.

The scan range should be set a little larger than actually needed to prevent these problems. When real-time

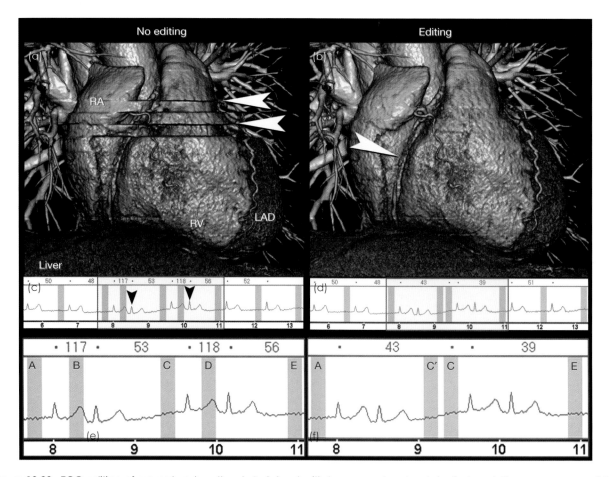

Figure 18.20 ECG editing of premature heartbeat. A dataset with two premature beats is displayed. The appearance of the dataset before and after ECG editing is displayed with an anterior view using three-dimensional volume rendering (a) and (b). The premature beats cause a complete misregistration of the stacks of images (arrowheads in (a)), while after editing the spatial relationship is restored and the chronic total occlusion of the right coronary artery becomes more clearly visible (arrowhead in (b)). The corresponding ECG signals are displayed in (c) and (d). The premature beats (black arrowheads in (c)) in the blue box are the targets for ECG editing. The software generally uses all R waves to determine the temporal windows (A–E in (e)). This causes the temporal windows to fall in the very short diastolic phase just before the premature beat (B and D in (e)). This phase does not match with the others (A, C and E in (e)). After ECG editing (d) and (f), the temporal windows located in the diastolic phase that preceded the premature beats (B and D in (e)) are deleted (f), and an additional temporal window (C' in (f)) is added to provide the software with enough information to reconstruct one image between two adjacent temporal windows. RA, right atrium; LAD, left anterior descending; LV, left ventricle; RV, right ventricle

display of the actual position of the table is available, the operator should use a longer scan range and stop the scan when the entire heart has been scanned.

VESSEL ENHANCEMENT

A high vascular enhancement is required to improve the visualization of small vessels (Table 18.1). In some cases the enhancement will not be satisfactory, regardless of an optimal intravenous administration protocol.

Poor vascular enhancement can occur when the patient has an extremely fast venoarterial circulation time or the position of the region of interest in the ascending aorta, that is used to trigger the bolus tracking, is not optimal (Figure 18.23). Other causes of poor enhancement are usually related to suboptimal contrast material administration. When the great vessels of the thorax do not show contrast visualization a technical failure of the contrast material administration procedure is usually the cause.

IMAGE QUALITY

An image is of high quality when the contours of the objects are sharp and it is easy to recognize the vessel contours and coronary plaques (Table 18.1).

To obtain sharp images the residual motion should be minimized, enhancement inside the lumen should be high (≈ 300 HU) and image noise should be minimized.

Image noise may not be evenly distributed in the data set when a premature heartbeat occurs and the prospective tube current modulation is active, which causes modulation to be activated during the diastolic phase (Figure 18.24). To prevent this artifact it is recommended that the ECG of the patient prior to the scan and during a test apnea be carefully observed to check for the presence of premature heartbeats. When premature heartbeats are present the operator should switch off the prospective tube current modulation.

CLASSIFICATIONS

The classification of artifacts in coronary CT can be based on the physics that creates the artifact, on the source of the artifact, or on the appearance of the artifact. A pragmatic approach would be to follow a 'chronological' classification. This implies that the sequence of the scan procedure is followed and the artifacts that are generated in each phase are explained. When available, solutions and practical advice are given to compensate or prevent the occurrence of the respective artifacts.

In Table 18.1 the various artifacts are summarized with reasons why the problems occur, what these problems cause and how they can be resolved, all of which is followed by practical advice.

CONCLUSION

Finally, one should be aware that artifacts are always present in CT imaging, related to the basics of the CT technique, while in cardiac CT imaging there are the additional cardiac contraction motion artifacts. It is expected that newer scanners with improved spatial and temporal resolution, and that more refined reconstruction algorithms and, eventually, different hardware resolutions will minimize the impact of artifacts in coronary CT imaging.

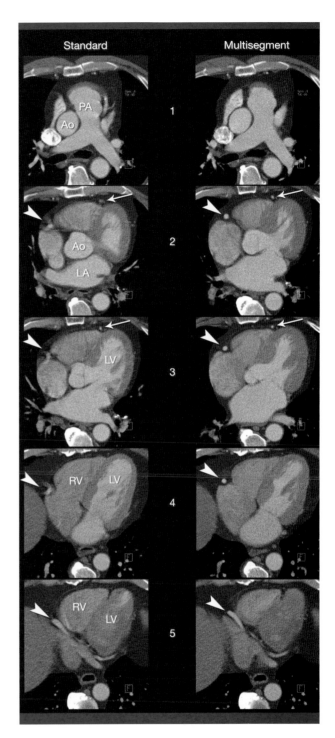

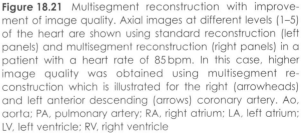

Figure 18.21 Multisegment reconstruction with improvement of image quality. Axial images at different levels (1–5) of the heart are shown using standard reconstruction (left panels) and multisegment reconstruction (right panels) in a patient with a heart rate of 85 bpm. In this case, higher image quality was obtained using multisegment reconstruction which is illustrated for the right (arrowheads) and left anterior descending (arrows) coronary artery. Ao, aorta; PA, pulmonary artery; RA, right atrium; LA, left atrium; LV, left ventricle; RV, right ventricle

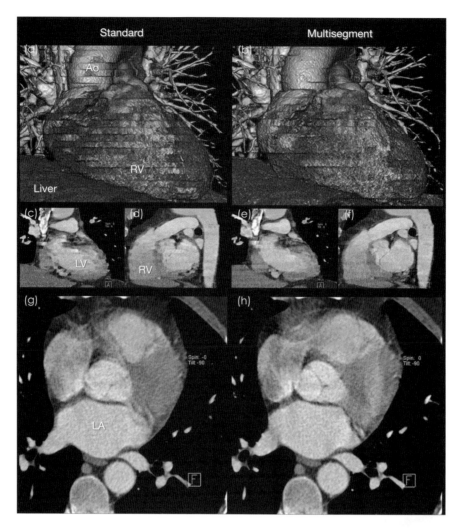

Figure 18.22 Multisegment reconstruction without significant improvement of image quality. Image quality did not significantly improve using multisegment reconstruction (right panels) when compared with that of standard reconstruction (left panels) in a patient with a mean heart rate of 92 bpm. Panels (a) and (b) are volume-rendered images showing better delineation of the left ventricle (LV) using multisegment reconstruction, which is also the case on the multiplanar-reconstructed images (c)–(f). However, the coronary angiographic image quality did not significantly improve using multisegment reconstruction which is illustrated on the axial images (g) and (h). Ao, aorta; LA, left atrium; RV, right ventricle

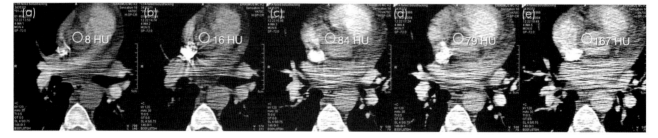

Figure 18.23 Failed bolus tracking. The circle highlights the region of interest which is positioned within the ascending aorta. Using a bolus tracking technique, scans are made at the same level to monitor the arrival of contrast material within the ascending aorta (a)–(e). These scans are not made during apnea and the position of the ascending aorta can differ within the monitoring scans. In this case, the region of interest was moved out of the region of the ascending aorta in several scans (c) and (d). Therefore, the arrival of the contrast material was not accurately detected and the angiography scan was started too late

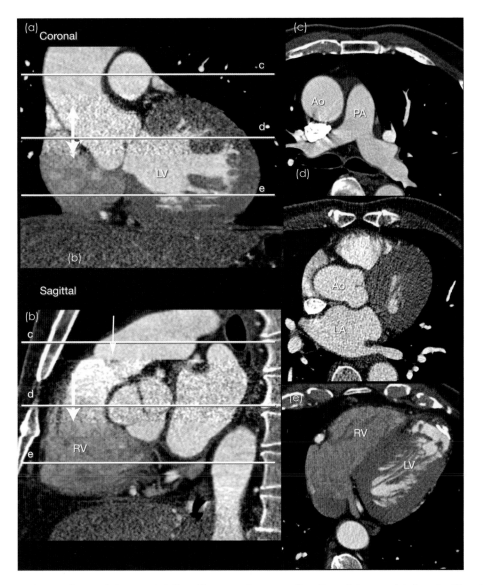

Figure 18.24 Incorrect use of X-ray tube modulation. The use of prospective X-ray tube modulation significantly reduces the radiation exposure during CT coronary angiography. However, this technique should not be used in patients with arrhythmia, because this can result in inaccurate synchronization timing and, consequently, a lower radiation output during the important diastolic phase. The effect of inaccurate tube modulation on image quality is clearly visible on the coronal (a) and sagittal (b) images (illustrated by the arrow) which was caused by a premature beat during the CT scan. High-quality axial images are shown at the levels with correct timing of the tube modulation (c)–(e), whereas image quality suffers from noise at the level of incorrect timing (d). Ao, aorta; PA, pulmonary artery; LA, left atrium; LV, left ventricle; RV, right ventricle

REFERENCES

1. Morgan CL. Basic Principles of Computed Tomography. Baltimore: University Park Press, 1983

2. Nieman K, Cademartiri F, Lemos PA, et al. Reliable noninvasive coronary angiography with fast submillimeter multislice spiral computed tomography. Circulation 2002; 106: 2051–4

3. Ropers D, Baum U, Pohle K, et al. Detection of coronary artery stenoses with thin-slice multi-detector row spiral computed tomography and multiplanar reconstruction. Circulation 2003; 107: 664–6

4. Hu H, He HD, Foley WD, Fox SH. Four multidetector-row helical CT: image quality and volume coverage speed. Radiology 2000; 215: 55–62

CHAPTER 19

Contrast enhancement in coronary angiography

To perform computed tomography (CT) coronary angiography it is mandatory to obtain prominent vascular enhancement. Because contrast material is administered intravenously, the scan has to be performed during the first pass of contrast material within the vessels of interest, which is usually defined as the arterial phase of contrast passage[1].

The presence of contrast material inside an artery generates a high contrast between the arterial lumen and the adjacent structures (including vessel wall, perivascular soft tissues and neighboring veins). Appropriate arterial enhancement significantly improves the quality of image post-processing and increases confidence in the evaluation of coronary abnormalities. To obtain the optimal arterial enhancement for

the purpose of CT coronary angiography several issues need to be addressed.

BOLUS GEOMETRY

Bolus geometry is the pattern of enhancement represented as a time–density curve (Figure 19.1) in a given vessel after the administration of a bolus of contrast material. Optimal bolus geometry is characterized by a rectangular shape, with a steep rise of the curve to a maximum plateau which lasts a little longer than the CT time followed by a steep descent. However, such bolus geometry cannot be achieved in clinical practice. Instead, the bolus geometry observed *in vivo* is charac-

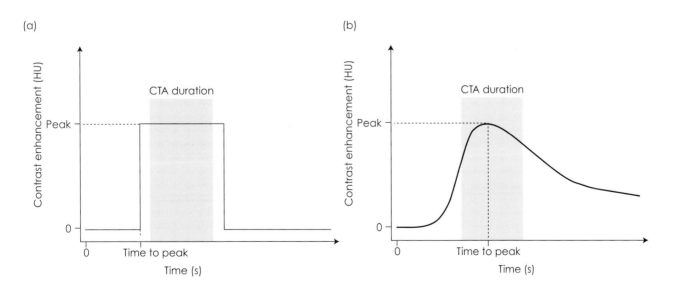

Figure 19.1 Bolus geometry. (a) Optimal bolus geometry. Enhancement in the vessel of interest rises with a very steep slope up to the peak, and then remains steady for the whole plateau, which ideally is a little longer than the scan time. (b) Actual bolus geometry. In actual bolus geometry there is a slow increase in vascular enhancement up to a peak. Then, the enhancement starts to drop. No real plateau of enhancement occurs. CTA, computed tomography angiography

terized by a slow increase of the curve, a delay to reach the peak rather than a plateau, and is followed by a slow decrease of enhancement. It is important to recognize this and that the timing and duration of CT scanning should be synchronized to the timing and duration of the actual bolus geometry.

Optimization of the bolus geometry

Actual bolus geometry is influenced by several parameters that are patient related such as age, body weight and cardiac output[2–8] or are related to the modality of contrast-material administration, which are operator controlled. Contrast-injection parameters and synchronization of bolus geometry and CT scan timing play a significant role in the actual bolus geometry.

CONTRAST-MATERIAL INJECTION PARAMETERS

Contrast-material injection parameters are contrast-material volume, injection rate and iodine concentration (Figure 19.2).

Contrast-material volume

An increase in contrast-injection volume produces an increase in arterial enhancement. However, there is also a delay in the time to peak of maximum enhancement[9–11] (Figure 19.2a).

It is of note that higher patient weight is associated with poorer performance of the contrast administration protocol. This is partly owing to the larger blood pool of heavier patients, which decreases the contrast enhancement, and partly to the higher attenuation of X-rays, which decreases the signal to noise ratio. It is recommended that the volume of contrast material be increased by 20–25% when the patient's weight is more than 90 kg.

Contrast-injection rate

An increase in injection rate produces an increase in arterial enhancement. In addition, there is an earlier peak of maximum enhancement[7,9,10,12–14] (Figure 19.2b).

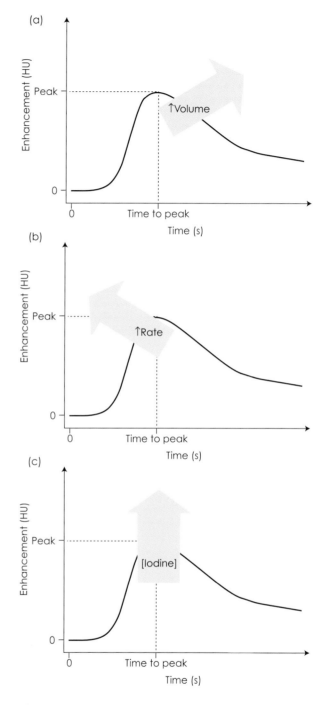

Figure 19.2 Injection parameters. (a) Effect of contrast-material volume. An increase in the volume of contrast material produces a concomitant increase in the peak of maximum enhancement and a delay in the time to peak. (b) Effect of contrast-material rate. An increase in the rate of contrast-material injection produces a concomitant increase in the peak of maximum enhancement and an anticipation of the time to peak. (c) Effect of contrast-material iodine concentration. An increase in contrast-material iodine concentration produces an increase in the peak of maximum enhancement without any influence on the time to peak

However, the effects of the increase in the injection rate are limited because a higher rate of injection into a cubital vein may be associated with a higher chance of contrast material extravasation. Therefore, in practice the injection rate used ranges between 4 and 5 ml/s.

Contrast-material iodine concentration

An increase in the iodine concentration of the contrast material produces an increase in arterial enhancement[10,15], while the time to peak of maximum enhancement remains unaffected (Figure 19.2c). It is of note that owing to the higher viscosity of compounds with a high iodine concentrations they should be heated to 38°C before injection. Also, a higher iodine concentration is associated with a higher chance of renal dysfunction.

It has been suggested that multiphasic protocols using varying injection rates during the injection of contrast material should improve the homogeneity of the plateau of arterial enhancement[8,16–19]. However, modern 16-row multislice scanners have reduced the scan time to less than 20 s, thereby obviating the need for such protocols.

CONTRAST-MATERIAL SYNCHRONIZATION TECHNIQUES

Contrast-material synchronization techniques are fixed delay, test bolus and bolus tracking. With these techniques the operator tries to synchronize optimally the peak of maximum arterial enhancement with the CT angiography scan (Figure 19.3).

Fixed delay technique

A fixed delay between the start of intravenous administration of contrast material and the start of the scan is not optimal. The variability in the delay of peak maximum enhancement is substantial, mainly due to patient-related parameters (Figure 19.3a). For instance, in patients with impaired left ventricular function a delay of typically 18–20 s as occurs in normal situations is too short and will result in scanning of coronary arteries that are not yet enhanced.

Test bolus technique

The test bolus technique is based on the calculation of the transit time between the site of injection and the ascending aorta using a small volume of contrast material as a test bolus (10–15 ml)[1,6,7] (Figure 19.3b).

This technique has been demonstrated to be reliable; however, it is not perfect. It has been reported that there is a correlation between the delay calculated by means of the test bolus and a point on the up slope of the curve of bolus geometry, but no correlation with the peak of maximum enhancement[4,7].

Bolus tracking technique

The bolus tracking technique is based on real-time monitoring of the arrival of contrast material in the ascending aorta. During the intravenous injection, the arrival of contrast material is monitored by dynamic acquisition of a single slice at the level of the ascending aorta. When a predetermined density threshold of enhancement is achieved within the lumen of the ascending aorta, the CT scan is automatically triggered[1] (Figure 19.3c).

The threshold used for optimal triggering of the scan is 100 HU above the baseline value of attenuation of the ascending aorta sampled in an non-enhanced premonitoring scan. Therefore, the actual value of attenuation that triggers the scan will vary between 50 and 100 HU.

The arrival of contrast material triggers the scan, and the table automatically moves to the previously set starting position; in the meantime breath-hold instructions are given to the patient. This step usually requires 4–5 s. The scan can then be started. Bolus tracking has been demonstrated to produce better results in terms of vascular enhancement when compared with other techniques[20–22].

OTHER PARAMETERS

Bolus chaser

In addition to the main parameters already discussed, there are additional measures that can improve the modality of administration and the use of contrast material in cardiac CT, such as bolus chaser. Bolus chaser is a volume of saline that is injected immediately after

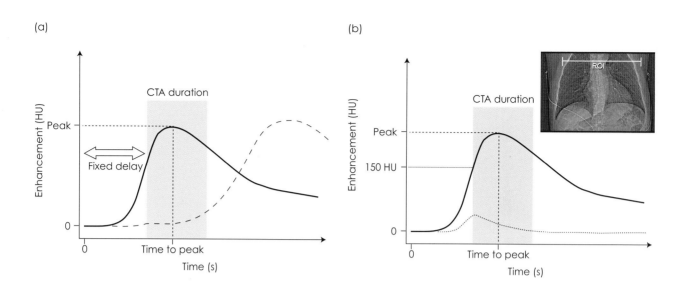

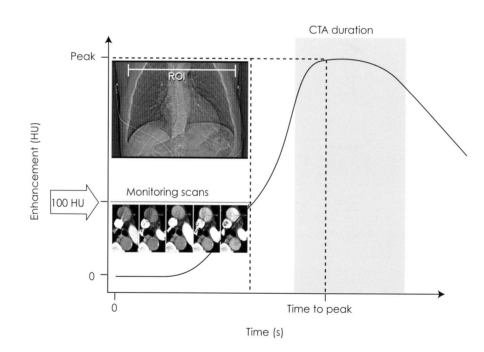

Figure 19.3 Synchronization techniques. (a) Fixed delay. The use of a fixed delay is very practical because it does not require any technical optimization; however, it is not appropriate in every patient. The major risk is that in a patient with slow venoarterial circulation, the scan is performed when the contrast material has not yet arrived in the coronary arteries (dashed line). (b) Test bolus. The use of a test bolus allows calculation of the transit time between the injection site (e.g. antecubital vein) and the ascending aorta. A period of 4–6 s should be added to the calculated delay in order to fit with the bolus geometry of the angiographic bolus. (c) Bolus tracking. The use of a real-time bolus tracking technique allows the delay to be tailored to each patient without the use of additional contrast material and it is based on the actual bolus geometry of the main angiographic bolus rather than on a smaller test bolus. During the injection of contrast material, a series of monitoring scans sample the enhancement in the ascending aorta, and when the trigger threshold is reached (+100 HU), the scan is automatically started after the 4 s that are necessary to give the patient breath-hold instructions. ROI, region of interest; CTA, computed tomography angiography

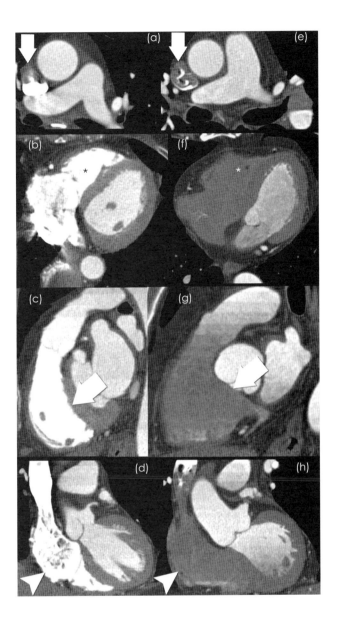

Figure 19.4 Effect of bolus chaser on bolus geometry. In the images a protocol with the same volume of contrast material is compared without (a)–(d) and with bolus chaser (e)–(h). Several different images are displayed to highlight the presence or reduction of vascular enhancement owing to the administration of bolus chaser. In (a) and (e) the two different protocols are compared in an axial image at the level of the ascending aorta and pulmonary artery. The superior vena cava at this level (arrows) is very bright in (a), where there is no bolus chaser, and is almost un-enhanced in (b), where a bolus chaser follows the main bolus. In (b) and (f) the two different protocols are compared in an axial image at a midventricular level. The right chambers of the heart are hyperdense (asterisk) (b) or hypodense (asterisk) (f) depending on the absence or presence of a bolus chaser. The same patterns are displayed in a sagittal plane passing through the right ventricle and pulmonary artery (arrows) (c) and (g), and in a coronal plane passing through the right ventricle and superior vena cava (arrowheads) (d) and (h)

the bolus of contrast material (Figure 19.4). Usually it is administered at the same rate as the contrast-material bolus. To administer a bolus chaser it is necessary to use either two parallel injectors or a single double-head injector[23,24]. The rationale behind the use of a bolus chaser is based on flushing of the contrast material after the end of the injection. With the bolus chaser the contrast material is pushed at a predetermined speed, while without it it slows down to the speed provided by the venous flow. The use of bolus chaser has been reported to provide benefits in terms of reduction of contrast-material volume and beam-hardening artifacts at the level of the thoracic outlet, superior vena cava and right atrium and ventricle[23,27], which is desirable for better evaluation of the right coronary artery.

Injection site and device

Usually a large and proximal antecubital vein is used for CT coronary angiography. An 18–20-gauge intravenous cannula allows the desired injection rate to be achieved without complications (e.g. vein rupture and contrast extravasation). We have found that in nearly all men an 18-gauge cannula can be inserted without much difficulty, while in women or overweight patients a 20-gauge cannula is easier.

NON-CORONARY STUDIES

In the evaluation of cardiac thrombi, cardiac/pericardial and mediastinal masses, and the visualization of cardiac veins, high vascular enhancement is not necessary and a lower injection rate with the same contrast-material volume will produce longer vascular enhancement. A delayed scan phase can be helpful depicting the pattern of vascularization of a cardiac mass. Cardiac veins can be visualized by simply increasing the scan delay by 10 s or by using a higher trigger threshold (e.g. 150–175 HU) in bolus tracking.

RECOMMENDATIONS

Adequate vascular enhancement is of paramount importance to the success of coronary CT angiography. The injection parameters and resulting synchronization protocols should be optimal (Table 19.1).

Table 19.1 Recommendations for contrast enhancement in CT coronary angiography

Parameters	Coronary CTA	Comment	Non-coronary CT	Comment
Injection				
Volume (ml)	100	increase when the scan range, and therefore the scan time, increases (e.g. CABG)	100	increase when the scan range, and therefore the scan time, increases (e.g. study of the entire thorax)
Rate (ml/s)	4	increase to 5 ml/s when scan time is below 15 s and the antecubital vein is large	3	a lower rate is preferable and allows longer enhancement
Iodine concentration (mg/ml)	350–400	preferably 400 mg/ml	300–400	—
Synchronization				
Fixed delay (s)	18–20	increase of 5–10 s in patients with reduced cardiac output	18–20	increase of 5–10 s in patients with reduced cardiac output
Test bolus				
volume (ml)	15–20	or 15–20% of the main contrast-material bolus	15–20	or 15–20% of the main contrast-material bolus
rate (ml/s)	4		4	
delay (s)	TT + 4–6 s		TT + 4–6 s	
Bolus tracking				
ROI	ascending aorta	positioned in the center of the vessel as seen on axial premonitoring images	ascending aorta	positioned in the center of the vessel as seen on axial premonitoring images
threshold (HU)	+100	no less than 75 HU to avoid anticipated triggering from beam-hardening artifacts in the superior vena cava	+100	no less than 75 HU to avoid anticipated triggering from beam-hardening artifacts in the superior vena cava
Others				
Bolus chaser				not required
volume (ml)	40	or 35–40% of the contrast-material bolus	—	—
rate (ml/s)	4	or same rate as contrast material	—	—
CM administration				
site	antecubital	recommended because it reduces the chances of contrast-material extravasation and the diffusion of contrast material in collateral venous pathways	antecubital	recommended because it reduces the chances of contrast-material extravasation and the diffusion of contrast material in collateral venous pathways
side	right	recommended because the right subclavian and innominate veins are not crossing the aortic arch	right	recommended because the right subclavian and innominate veins are not crossing the aortic arch

CABG, coronary artery bypass graft; CM, contrast material; CT, computed tomography; CTA, computed tomography angiography; ROI, region of interest; TT, transit time

In clinical practice, 16-row (or higher) multislice CT scanners require an injection volume of approximately 100 ml for sufficient enhancement during the entire duration of the CT angiography scan. Because the recommended injection rate is 4 ml/s, the contrast-material administration time will be 25 s, which is a little longer than the average scan time.

The ideal iodine concentration for coronary CT angiography should be 350 mg/ml or more. With this concentration, high vascular enhancement can be pro-duced without a corresponding increase in injection rate. When using a high iodine concentration contrast material (monomeric ≥ 350 mg/ml or dimeric 320 mg/ml), it should be noted that, because of their high viscosity, they must be administered only after appropriate heating at 38°C.

The optimal technique for contrast-material synchronization is bolus tracking, which is available on current multislice CT scanners with cardiac imaging capabilities. The trigger threshold of attenuation for the region of interest in the ascending aorta should be chosen around +100 HU. A lower threshold will be too sensitive to beam-hardening artifacts in the superior vena cava resulting in early triggering with scan failure.

The test bolus technique can also be used, but better vascular enhancement is achieved by the addition of 4–6 s to delay the transit time of the test bolus between the injection site and ascending aorta.

REFERENCES

1. Cademartiri F, van der Lugt A, Luccichenti G, et al. Parameters affecting bolus geometry in CTA: a review. J Comput Assist Tomogr 2002; 26: 598–607

2. Handlin LR, Kindred LH, Beauchamp GD, et al. Reversible left ventricular dysfunction after subarachnoid hemorrhage. Am Heart J 1993; 126: 235–40

3. Kono T, Morita H, Kuroiwa T, et al. Left ventricular wall motion abnormalities in patients with subarachnoid hemorrhage: neurogenic stunned myocardium. J Am Coll Cardiol 1994; 24: 636–40

4. van Hoe L, Marchal G, Baert AL, et al. Determination of scan delay time in spiral CT-angiography: utility of a test bolus injection. J Comput Assist Tomogr 1995; 19: 216–20

5. Bae KT, Heiken JP, Brink JA. Aortic and hepatic contrast medium enhancement at CT. Part II. Effect of reduced cardiac output in a porcine model. Radiology 1998; 207: 657–62

6. Nakajima Y, Yoshimine T, Yoshida H, et al. Computerized tomography angiography of ruptured cerebral aneurysms: factors affecting time to maximum contrast concentration. J Neurosurg 1998; 88: 663–9

7. Platt JF, Reige KA, Ellis JH. Aortic enhancement during abdominal CT angiography: correlation with test injections, flow rates, and patient demographics. Am J Roentgenol 1999; 172: 53–6

8. Fleischmann D, Rubin GD, Bankier AA, Hittmair K. Improved uniformity of aortic enhancement with customized contrast medium injection protocols at CT angiography. Radiology 2000; 214: 363–71

9. Garcia P, Genin G, Bret PM, et al. Hepatic CT enhancement: effect of the rate and volume of contrast medium injection in an animal model. Abdom Imaging 1999; 24: 597–603

10. Han JK, Kim AY, Lee KY, et al. Factors influencing vascular and hepatic enhancement at CT: experimental study on injection protocol using a canine model. J Comput Assist Tomogr 2000; 24: 400–6

11. Yamashita Y, Komohara Y, Takahashi M, et al. Abdominal helical CT: evaluation of optimal doses of intravenous contrast material – a prospective randomized study. Radiology 2000; 216: 718–23

12. Bae KT, Heiken JP, Brink JA. Aortic and hepatic peak enhancement at CT: effect of contrast medium injection rate – pharmacokinetic analysis and experimental porcine model. Radiology 1998; 206: 455–64

13. Kim T, Murakami T, Takahashi S, et al. Effects of injection rates of contrast material on arterial phase hepatic CT. Am J Roentgenol 1998; 171: 429–32

14. Luboldt W, Straub J, Seemann M, et al. Effective contrast use in CT angiography and dual-phase hepatic CT performed with a subsecond scanner. Invest Radiol 1999; 34: 751–60

15. Bluemke DA, Fishman EK, Anderson JH. Effect of contrast concentration on abdominal enhancement in the rabbit: spiral computed tomography evaluation. Acad Radiol 1995; 2: 226–31

16. Hittmair K, Fleischmann D. Accuracy of predicting and controlling time-dependent aortic enhancement from a test bolus injection. J Comput Assist Tomogr 2001; 25: 287–94

17. Fleischmann D, Hittmair K. Mathematical analysis of arterial enhancement and optimization of bolus geometry for CT angiography using the discrete Fourier transform. J Comput Assist Tomogr 1999; 23: 474–84

18. Bae KT, Heiken JP, Brink JA. Aortic and hepatic contrast medium enhancement at CT. Part I. Prediction with a computer model. Radiology 1998; 207: 647–55

19. Bae KT, Tran HQ, Heiken JP. Multiphasic injection method for uniform prolonged vascular enhancement at CT angiography: pharmacokinetic analysis and experimental porcine model. Radiology 2000; 216: 872–80

20. Kopka L, Rodenwaldt J, Fischer U, et al. Dual-phase helical CT of the liver: effects of bolus tracking and different volumes of contrast material. Radiology 1996; 201: 321–6

21. Kirchner J, Kickuth R, Laufer U, et al. Optimized enhancement in helical CT: experiences with a real-time bolus tracking system in 628 patients. Clin Radiol 2000; 55: 368–73

22. Cademartiri F, Nieman K, van der Lugt A, et al. IV contrast administration for CT coronary angiography on a 16-multidetector-row helical CT scanner: test bolus vs. bolus tracking. Radiology 2004; in press

23. Haage P, Schmitz-Rode T, Hubner D, et al. Reduction of contrast material dose and artifacts by a saline flush using a double power injector in helical CT of the thorax. Am J Roentgenol 2000; 174: 1049–53

24. Cademartiri F, Mollet N, van der Lugt A, et al. Non-invasive 16-row multislice CT coronary angiography: usefulness of saline chaser. Eur Radiol 2004; 14: 178–83

25. Hopper KD, Mosher TJ, Kasales CJ, et al. Thoracic spiral CT: delivery of contrast material pushed with injectable saline solution in a power injector. Radiology 1997; 205: 269–71

26. Sadick M, Lehmann KJ, Diehl SJ, et al. [Bolus tracking and NaCl bolus in biphasic spiral CT of the abdomen]

Bolustriggerung und NaCl-Bolus bei der biphasischen Spiral-CT des Abdomens. Rofo Fortschr Geb Rontgenstr Neuen Bildgeb Verfahr 1997; 167: 371–6

27. Bader TR, Prokesch RW, Grabenwoger F. Timing of the hepatic arterial phase during contrast-enhanced computed tomography of the liver: assessment of normal values in 25 volunteers. Invest Radiol 2000; 35: 486–92

CHAPTER 20

The future

Coronary imaging remains the ultimate challenge for any non-invasive imaging technique. Although great strides have been made in CT coronary angiography many problems remain to be resolved before CT coronary imaging becomes accepted as a reliable substitute for invasive coronary angiography (Table 20.1). The coronary vessels have small dimensions which require high spatial resolution, ideally isotropic imaging. Cardiac contraction causes significant motion artifacts, in particular at high heart rates; however, sufficient temporal resolution should diminish this problem. Severe local coronary calcification may obscure interpretation of the underlying coronary lumen, and the blooming artifact of calcium, due to beam hardening and partial voluming, often leads to overestimation of the severity of an associated coronary stenosis. Increased spatial resolution should reduce this problem; however, in addition, specific algorithms that may partly reduce the calcium-induced artifacts should be helpful. A significant problem is the high X-ray radiation exposure of spiral CT scanners (Table 20.2). Effective doses for men and women range from 7.6 to 13 mSv for four-slice MSCT scanners, while the radiation exposure of 16-slice MSCT scanners is currently not known, but is expected to be even higher than that from four-slice MSCT scanners. The effective dose can be reduced by approximately 50% when an ECG-dependent dose-modulation protocol is used, so that the full radiation dose is only given during the diastolic cardiac phase with acquisition of data for image reconstruction, and a much lower dose is given during the systolic phase (data not used for image reconstruction).

The current MSCT technology with good diagnostic performance in a selected population (younger patients with stable heart rhythm and low heart rate) induces high hopes that the technique may become a reliable alternative to invasive diagnostic coronary angiography. This is further strengthened by the introduction of a 64-

Table 20.1 Future challenges of multislice CT (MSCT) coronary imaging

Problem	Solution
Small vessels	higher spatial resolution
Cardiac motion artifacts	higher temporal resolution at least 100 ms (ideally 50 ms)
Coronary calcification	increased spatial resolution (isotropic voxels), dedicated algorithms
Radiation exposure	ECG-triggered X-ray modulation
Irregular heart rhythm	acquisition during one heart cycle
Clinical reliability	MSCT tested in a wide range of populations with different prevalences of disease including elderly patients (higher likelihood of calcium) and in various clinical situations
Visual assessment	quantification algorithms

ECG, electrocardiogram

slice MSCT scanner, which has a significantly improved spatial resolution (Figure 20.1). Before embracing MSCT as an alternative to diagnostic invasive coronary angiography, the clinical role of MSCT coronary angiography must be assessed in a broad range of patient populations in various clinical situations. The advantages and disadvantages of CT coronary imaging compared to invasive diagnostic coronary angiography are

listed in Table 20.3. Future potential applications of CT coronary imaging (Table 20.4) may significantly improve the ability to evaluate coronary atherosclerosis in various clinical situations, including replacement of established invasive coronary angiographic indications and new applications exclusively related to the non-invasive nature of CT coronary angiography, which also allows coronary plaque imaging.

Table 20.2 CT radiation exposure

	EBCT		Four-slice MSCT			16-slice MSCT
	CAC scoring triggered	CTCA triggered	CTCA scoring triggered	CAC scoring gated	CTA triggered	
Exposure time (s)	0.1	0.1	0.33–0.36	0.5	0.5	—
Collimation N x T	1 x 3	1 x 3	4 x 2.5	4 x 2.5	4 x 1–1.25	—
Table feed (mm)	3	2	10	3.75	1.5–1.9	—
Effective dose (mSv)	0.7	1.1	1.0	2.6–4.1	9.3–11.3	—

EBCT, electron-beam CT; CAC, coronary artery calcium; CTCA, CT coronary angiography

Table 20.3 Comparison of invasive diagnostic coronary angiography with multislice CT (MSCT)

	Diagnostic coronary angiography	MSCT
Patient friendly	invasive	non-invasive
Facility	day care	out-patient clinic
Serious complication	<0.1%	very rare
Reading examination	cardiologist	cardiologist/radiologist
Costs of procedure	high	low
Procedural time (min)	30	10
Post-processing time (min)	0	20
Throughput	low	high
Performance investigation	cardiologist/nurse/technician	technician
Resolution	high	acceptable
Installation costs	no difference	no difference
Obstruction estimation	QCA	visual
Non-obstructive plaque	–	+
Calcified plaque	+	+++
Collaterals	high	minimal
Motion artifacts	none	unacceptable at high R-to-R interval
Radiation exposure (mSv)	6–8	8–10
Availability	worldwide	limited

QCA, quantitative coronary angiography

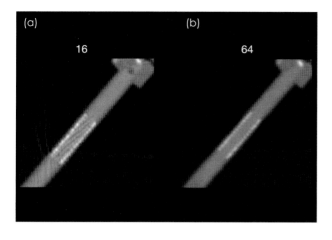

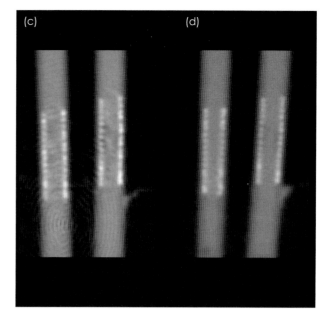

Figure 20.1 (a) and (c) *Ex vivo* stent imaging with 16-slice CT scanner: stent strut artifacts are clearly visible. (b) and (d) *Ex vivo* stent imaging with 64-slice CT scanner: the stent strut artifacts are smaller compared with those produced by the 16-slice CT scanner

Table 20.5 MSCT comprehensive cardiac imaging

Coronary artery lumen

Obstructions/occlusions

Coronary artery wall
    Plaques
        non-calcified
        calcified
        mixed

LV function
    Wall motion/ejection fraction

LV perfusion
    Functional ischemia

LV, left ventrical

MSCT coronary imaging has enormous potential, and volumetric acquisition of the entire heart in one breath hold may, in the future, permit comprehensive cardiac imaging including assessment of the coronary lumen, coronary plaques and left ventricular function (Table 20.5 and Figures 20.1–4).

CONCLUSION

The technique of non-invasive CT coronary imaging represents a major advance in the evaluation of coronary atherosclerosis in clinical practice.

Table 20.4 Potential applications of MSCT coronary imaging

Evaluation of chest pain in patients with atypical chest pain and an equivocal stress test

Evaluation of coronary anomalies

Alternative to invasive coronary angiography preceding percutaneous coronary intervention (PCI) in hospitals without PCI facilities

Early detection of atherosclerosis in high-risk individuals

Evaluation of coronary atherosclerosis in asymptomatic patients with known coronary artery disease

Coronary risk evaluation in patients undergoing major non-cardiac surgery

Evaluation of CAD in non-ischemic patients scheduled for aortic or mitral valve operations

Evaluation of chest pain at emergency department

Evaluation of efficacy of thrombolytic treatment in ST segment elevation acute myocardial infarction

Evaluation of post-bypass surgery patients

Evaluation of in-stent restenosis after percutaneous stent implantation

Evaluation of lifestyle, dietary or pharmacological interventions on progression/regression of coronary atherosclerosis

CAD, coronary artery disease

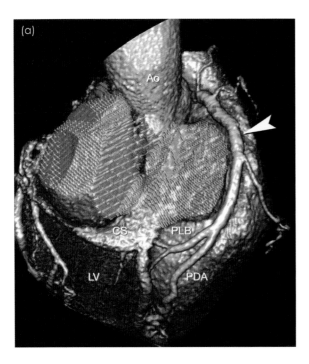

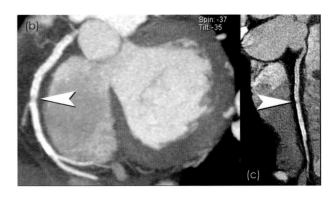

Figure 20.2a Three-dimensional volume-rendered image of the right coronary artery in which stents have been implanted (arrowhead). (a) MIP. (b) shows the extension and configuration of the stented segments. At the level of the arrowhead (b) there is a gap between the stents, also shown in the curved reconstruction ((C), arrowhead). The right coronary artery shows no signs of in-stent restenosis. CS, coronary sinus; LV, left ventricle; PDA, posterior descending coronary artery; PLB, postero-lateral branch

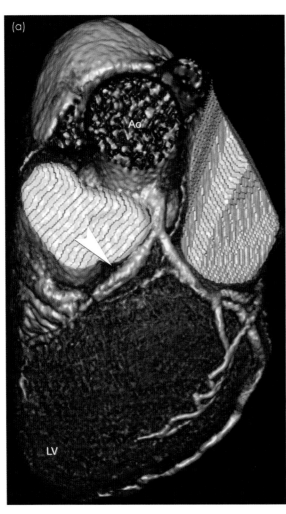

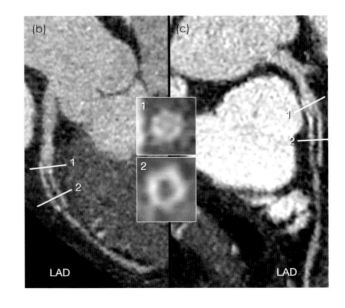

Figure 20.2b A 64-slice CT with coronary stents in LAD (arrowhead) The curved reconstructions performed in orthogonal planes in (b) and (c) show an area of lower density (indicative of neo-intimal hyperplasia) inside the lumen of the stent. The cross-sections performed at the level of the proximal end of the stent (1) and at the level of the middle portion (2) show patent and occluded stent, respectively. The segments distal of the occluded coronary stent are filled by collaterals. LAD, left anterior descending artery; LV, left ventricle

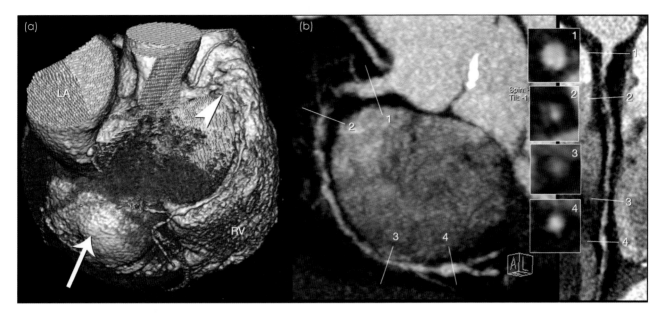

Figure 20.3a Visualization of coronary plaques with 64-slice CT (right coronary artery). (a), the right coronary artery with atherosclerotic involvement of the entire vessel. The left ventricle shows a large area of thinning in the inferior wall due to a previous infarction (thin arrow). The MIP (b) and the curved reconstruction (c) show the diffusely diseased right coronary artery. Cross-sections along the vessel (1–4) demonstrate the different degrees of lumen stenosis and coronary wall thickening. LA, left atrium; RV, right ventricle

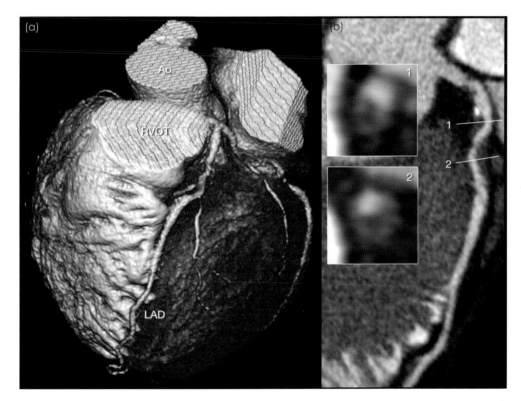

Figure 20.3b Visualization of coronary plaques with 64-slice CT (left anterior descending coronary artery). A diffusely diseased left anterior descending coronary artery is displayed (a). The curved reconstruction (b) shows the presence of large predominantly non-calcified plaques in the proximal left anterior descending coronary artery. The cross-sections (1–2) show positive remodeling. Ao, ascending aorta; LAD, left anterior descending; RVOT, right ventricle outflow tract

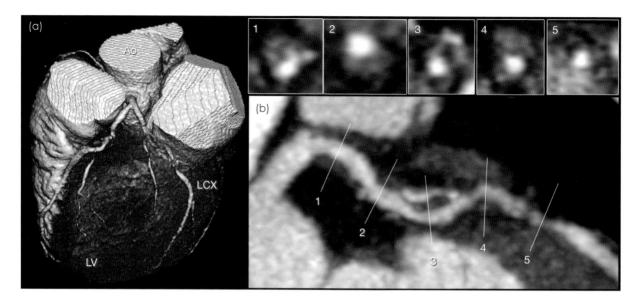

Figure 20.3c Visualization of coronary plaques with 64-slice CT (left circumflex coronary artery). A diffusely diseased left circumflex coronary artery is displayed (a). The curved reconstruction (b) shows the presence of large predominantly non-calcified plaques in the proximal left circumflex coronary artery. The cross-sections (1–5) show positive remodeling. Ao, ascending aorta; LCX, left circumflex coronary artery; LV, left ventricle

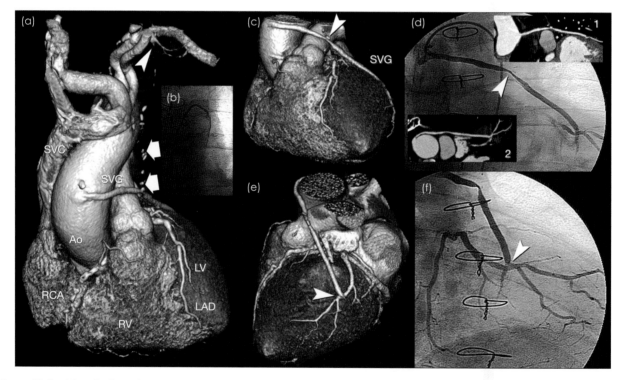

Figure 20.4a Visualization of the thoracic cardiovascular system in patient with previous CABG with 64-slice CT. Specifications: 100 ml of intravenous contrast material and a scan of 18–20 seconds with a voxel size of 0.4 mm3. The left internal mammary artery is visible only at its origin ((a), arrowhead) while the remaining segments are occluded ((a), thick arrows). A conventional coronary angiography confirmed these findings (b). The single saphenous vein graft was patent but showed a stenosis in the middle segment (arrowhead in (c)–(d)) both evident at three-dimensional volume rendering (c) and at curved reconstructions (1–2 in (d)). The conventional coronary angiography confirmed these findings (d). The distal anastomosis of the saphenous vein graft (arrowhead in (E)–(F)) was patent. Ao, ascending aorta; LAD, left anterior descending coronary artery; LV, left ventricle; RV, right ventricle; SVC, superior vena cava; SVG, saphenous vein graft; CABG, coronary artery bypass grafting

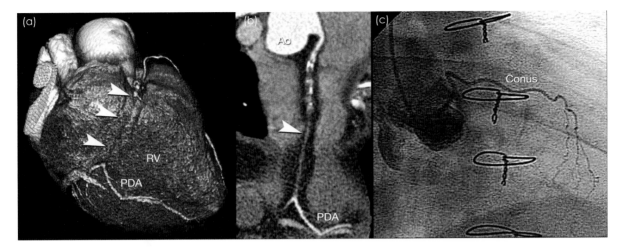

Figure 20.4b MSCT of the RCA of same patient. The right coronary artery is occluded ((a)–(b), arrowheads) which is confirmed by conventional coronary angiography (c). PDA, posterior descending coronary artery; RV, right ventricle

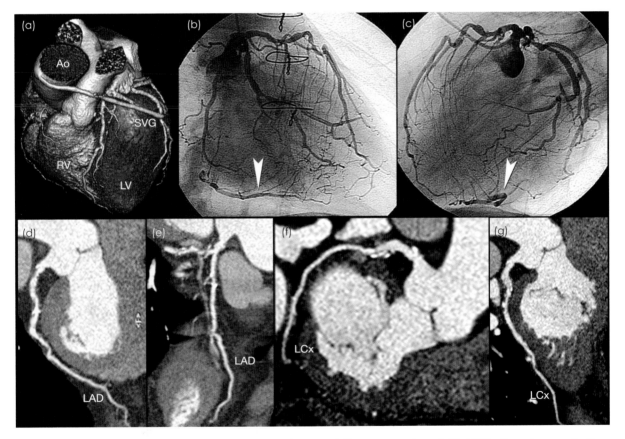

Figure 20.4c MSCT of the left coronary artery of same patient. The left coronary artery, (LAD, LCX) although severely diseased does not have a significant lumen stenosis ((a), (d)–(g)), as was confirmed by conventional coronary angiography ((b),(c)). The posterior descending artery is filled by collaterals from the left coronary artery (arrowhead in (b)–(c)). Ao, ascending aorta; LAD, left anterior descending coronary artery; LCx, left circumflex coronary artery; LV, left ventricle; RV, right ventricle; SVG, saphenous vein graft

BIBLIOGRAPHY

Hunold P, Vogt FM, Schmermund A, et al. Radiation exposure during cardiac CT: effective doses at multi-detector row CT and electron-beam CT. Radiology 2003; 226: 145–52

Jakobs TF, Becker CR, Ohnesorge B, et al. Multislice helical CT of the heart with retrospective ECG gating: reduction of radiation exposure by ECG-controlled tube current modulation. Eur Radiol 2002; 12: 1081–6

Morin RL, Gerber TC, McCollough CH. Radiation dose in computed tomography of the heart. Circulation 2003; 107: 917–22

References

CLINICAL REFERENCES

1. Moshage WE, Achenbach S, Seese B, et al. Coronary artery stenoses: three-dimensional imaging with electrocardiographically triggered, contrast agent-enhanced, electron-beam CT. Radiology 1995; 196: 707–14

2. Achenbach S, Moshage W, Bachmann K. Detection of high-grade restenosis after PTCA using contrast-enhanced electron beam CT. Circulation 1997; 96: 2785–8

3. Nakanishi T, Ito K, Imazu M, et al. Evaluation of coronary artery stenoses using electron-beam CT and multiplanar reformation. J Comput Assist Tomogr 1997; 21: 121–7

4. Achenbach S, Moshage W, Ropers D, et al. Value of electron-beam computed tomography for the noninvasive detection of high-grade coronary-artery stenoses and occlusions. N Engl J Med 1998; 339: 1964–71

5. Rensing BJ, Bongaerts A, van Geuns RJ, et al. Intravenous coronary angiography by electron beam computed tomography: a clinical evaluation. Circulation 1998; 98: 2509–12

6. Reddy G, Chernoff DM, Adams JR, et al. Coronary artery stenoses: assessment with contrast-enhanced electron-beam CT and axial reconstructions. Radiology 1998; 208: 167–72

7. Schmermund A, Rensing BJ, Sheedy PF, et al. Intravenous electron-beam computed tomographic coronary angiography for segmental analysis of coronary artery stenoses. J Am Coll Cardiol 1998; 31: 1547–54

8. Budoff MJ, Oudiz RJ, Zalace CP, et al. Intravenous three-dimensional coronary angiography using contrast-enhanced electron beam computed tomography. Am J Cardiol 1999; 83: 840–5

9. Moshage W, Ropers D, Daniel WG, Achenbach S. [Noninvasive imaging of coronary arteries with electron beam tomography (EBCT).] Z Kardiol 2000; 89 (Suppl 1): 15–20

10. Achenbach S, Ropers D, Regenfus M, et al. Contrast enhanced electron beam computed tomography to analyse the coronary arteries in patients after acute myocardial infarction. Heart 2000; 84: 489–93

11. Achenbach S, Ulzheimer S, Baum U, et al. Noninvasive coronary angiography by retrospectively ECG-gated multislice spiral CT. Circulation 2000; 102: 2823–8

12. Nieman K, Oudkerk M, Rensing BJ, et al. Coronary angiography with multi-slice computed tomography. Lancet 2001; 357: 599–603

13. Achenbach S, Giesler T, Ropers D, et al. Detection of coronary artery stenoses by contrast-enhanced, retrospectively electrocardiographically-gated, multislice spiral computed tomography. Circulation 2001; 103: 2535–8

14. Knez A, Becker CR, Leber A, et al. Usefulness of multislice spiral computed tomography angiography for determination of coronary artery stenoses. Am J Cardiol 2001; 88: 1191–4

15. Schroeder S, Kopp AF, Baumbach A, et al. Noninvasive detection and evaluation of atherosclerotic coronary plaques with multislice computed tomography. J Am Coll Cardiol 2001; 37: 1430–5

16. Ropers D, Moshage W, Daniel WG, et al. Visualization of coronary artery anomalies and their anatomic course by contrast-enhanced electron beam tomography and three-dimensional reconstruction. Am J Cardiol 2001; 87: 193–7

17. Lu B, Zhuang N, Mao SS, et al. Image quality of three-dimensional electron beam coronary angiography. J Comput Assist Tomogr 2002; 26: 202–9

18. Vogl TJ, Abolmaali ND, Diebold T, et al. Techniques for the detection of coronary atherosclerosis: multidetector row CT coronary angiography. Radiology 2002; 223: 212–20

19. Kopp AF, Schröder S, Küttner A, et al. Non-invasive coronary angiography with high resolution multidetec-

tor-row computed tomography: results in 102 patients. Eur Heart J 2002; 23: 1714–25

20. Giesler T, Baum U, Ropers D, et al. Noninvasive visualization of coronary arteries using contrast-enhanced multidetector CT: influence of heart rate on image quality and stenosis detection. Am J Roentgenol 2002; 179: 911–16

21. Nieman K, Rensing BJ, van Geuns RJM, et al. Usefulness of multislice computed tomography for detecting obstructive coronary artery disease. Am J Cardiol 2002; 89: 913–18

22. Schroeder S, Kopp AF, Ohnesorge B, et al. Virtual coronary angioscopy using multislice computed tomography. Heart 2002; 87: 205–9

23. Nieman K, Cademartiri F, Lemos PA, et al. Reliable noninvasive coronary angiography with fast submillimeter multislice spiral computed tomography. Circulation 2002; 106: 2051–4

24. Nieman K, Rensing BJ, van Geuns RJ, et al. Non-invasive coronary angiography with multislice spiral computed tomography: impact of heart rate. Heart 2002; 88: 470–4

25. Ropers D, Gehling G, Pohle K, et al. Anomalous course of the left main or left anterior descending coronary artery originating from the right sinus of Valsalva. Identification of four common variations by electron beam tomography. Circulation 2002; 105: e42–e43

26. Dirksen MS, Bax JJ, de Roos A, et al. Usefulness of dynamic multislice computed tomography and left ventricular function in unstable angina pectoris and comparison with echocardiography. Am J Cardiol 2002; 90: 1157–60

27. Becker CR, Knez A, Leber A, et al. Detection of coronary artery stenoses with multislice helical CT angiography. J Comput Assist Tomogr 2002; 26: 750–5

28. Nieman K, Cademartiri F, Raaijmakers R, et al. Noninvasive angiographic evaluation of coronary stents with multi-slice spiral computed tomography. Herz 2003; 28: 136–42

29. Ropers D, Baum U, Pohle K, et al. Detection of coronary artery stenoses with thin-slice multi-detector row spiral computed tomography and multiplanar reconstruction. Circulation 2003; 107: 664–6

30. Achenbach S, Moselewski F, Ropers D, et al. Detection of calcified and noncalcified coronary atherosclerotic plaque by contrast-enhanced, submillimeter multidetector spiral computed tomography: a segment-based comparison with intravascular ultrasound. Circulation 2004; 109: 14–17. Epub 2003 Dec 22

31. Kuettner A, Kopp AF, Schroeder S, et al. Diagnostic accuracy of multidetector computed tomography coronary angiography in patients with angiographically proven coronary artery disease. J Am Coll Cardiol 2004; 43: 831–9

Technical references

1. Kalender WA, Seissler W, Klotz E, Vock P. Spiral volumetric CT with single-breath-hold technique, continuous transport, and continuous scanner rotation. Radiology 1990; 176: 181–3

2. Polacin A, Kalender WA, Marchal G. Evaluation of section sensitivity profiles and image noise in spiral CT. Radiology 1992; 185: 29–35

3. Kalender WA, Polacin A, Suss C. A comparison of conventional and spiral CT: an experimental study on the detection of spherical lesions. J Comput Assist Tomogr 1994; 18: 167–76

4. Polacin A, Kalender WA, Brink J, Vannier MA. Measurement of slice sensitivity profiles in spiral CT. Med Phys 1994; 21: 133–40

5. Thomas PJ, McCollough CH, Ritman EL. An electron-beam CT approach for transvenous coronary arteriography. J Comput Assist Tomogr 1995; 19: 383–9

6. Detrano R, Hsiai T, Wang S, et al. Prognostic value of coronary calcification and angiographic stenoses in patients undergoing coronary angiography. J Am Coll Cardiol 1996; 27: 285–90

7. Uchino A, Kato A, Kudo S. CT angiography using electron-beam computed tomography (EBCT): a phantom study. Radiat Med 1997; 15: 273–6

8. Kachelriess M, Kalender WA. Electrocardiogram-correlated image reconstruction from subsecond spiral computed tomography scans of the heart. Med Phys 1998; 25: 2417–31

9. Shrimpton PC, Edyvean S. CT scanner dosimetry. Br J Radiol 1998; 71: 1–3

10. Klingenbeck-Regn K, Schaller S, Flohr T, et al. Subsecond multi-slice computed tomography: basics and applications. Eur J Radiol 1999; 31: 110–24

11. Hu H. Multislice helical CT: scan and reconstruction. Med Phys 1999; 26: 5–18

12. Kalender WA, Wolf H, Suess C. Dose reduction in CT by anatomically adapted tube current modulation. II. Phantom measurements. Med Phys 1999; 26: 2248–53

13. Kalender WA, Wolf H, Suess C, et al. Dose reduction in CT by on-line tube current control: principles and validation on phantoms and cadavers. Eur Radiol 1999; 9: 323–8

14. Kalender WA, Schmidt B, Zankl M, Schmidt M. A PC program for estimating organ dose and effective dose

values in computed tomography. Eur Radiol 1999; 9: 555–62

15. Gies M, Kalender WA, Wolf H, Suess C. Dose reduction in CT by anatomically adapted tube current modulation. I. Simulation studies. Med Phys 1999; 26: 2235–47

16. Kachelriess M, Ulzheimer S, Kalender WA. ECG-correlated imaging of the heart with subsecond multislice spiral CT. IEEE Trans Med Imaging 2000; 19: 888–901

17. Mao SS, Lu B, Oudiz RJ, et al. Coronary artery motion in electron beam tomography. J Comput Assist Tomogr 2000; 24: 253–8

18. Achenbach S, Ropers D, Holle J, et al. In-plane coronary arterial motion velocity: measurement with electron beam CT. Radiology 2000; 216: 457–63

19. Kachelriess M, Ulzheimer S, Kalender WA. ECG-correlated image reconstruction from subsecond multi-slice spiral CT scans of the heart. Med Phys 2000; 27: 1881–902

20. Hu H, He HD, Foley WD, Fox SH. Four multidetector-row helical CT: image quality and volume coverage speed. Radiology 2000; 215: 55–62

21. Wang G, Crawford CR, Kalender WA. Multirow detector and cone-beam spiral/helical CT. IEEE Trans Med Imaging 2000; 19: 817–21

22. McCollough CH, Bruesewitz MR, Daly TR, Zink FE. Motion artifacts in subsecond conventional CT and electron-beam CT: pictorial demonstration of temporal resolution. Radiographics 2000; 20: 1675–81

23. Ohnesorge B, Flohr T, Becker C, et al. Cardiac imaging by means of electrocardiographically gated multisection spiral CT: initial experience. Radiology 2000; 217: 564–71

24. Kachelriess M, Schaller S, Kalender WA. Advanced single-slice rebinning in cone-beam spiral CT. Med Phys 2000; 27: 754–72

25. Fuchs T, Krause J, Schaller S, et al. Spiral interpolation algorithms for multislice spiral CT part II: measurement and evaluation of slice sensitivity profiles and noise at a clinical multislice system. IEEE Trans Med Imaging 2000; 19: 835–47

26. Schaller S, Flohr T, Klingenbeck K, et al. Spiral interpolation algorithm for multislice spiral CT part I: theory. IEEE Trans Med Imaging 2000; 19: 822–34

27. Kopp AF, Schroeder S, Kuettner A, et al. Coronary arteries: retrospectively ECG-gated multi-detector row CT angiography with selective optimization of the image reconstruction window. Radiology 2001; 221: 683–8

28. Silverman PM, Kalender WA, Hazle JD. Common terminology for single and multislice helical CT. Am J Roentgenol 2001; 176: 1135–6

29. Hong C, Becker CR, Huber A, et al. ECG-gated reconstructed multi-detector row CT coronary angiography: effect of varying trigger delay on image quality. Radiology 2001; 220: 712–17

30. Becker CR, Kleffel T, Crispin A, et al. Coronary artery calcium measurement: agreement of multirow detector and electron beam CT. Am J Roentgenol 2001; 176: 1295–8

31. Jakobs TF, Becker CR, Ohnesorge B, et al. Multislice helical CT of the heart with retrospective ECG gating: reduction of radiation exposure by ECG-controlled tube current modulation. Eur Radiol 2002; 12: 1081–6

32. Kopp AF, Ohnesorge B, Becker C, et al. Reproducibility and accuracy of coronary calcium measurements with multi-detector row versus electron-beam CT. Radiology 2002; 225: 113–19

33. Hong C, Becker CR, Schoepf UJ, et al. Coronary artery calcium: absolute quantification in nonenhanced and contrast-enhanced multi-detector row CT studies. Radiology 2002; 223: 474–80

34. Ohnesorge B, Flohr T, Fischbach R, et al. Reproducibility of coronary calcium quantification in repeat examinations with retrospectively ECG-gated multisection spiral CT. Eur Radiol 2002; 12: 1532–40

35. Flohr T, Prokop M, Becker C, et al. A retrospectively ECG-gated multislice spiral CT scan and reconstruction technique with suppression of heart pulsation artifacts for cardio-thoracic imaging with extended volume coverage. Eur Radiol 2002; 12: 1497–503

36. Ulzheimer S, Kalender WA. Assessment of calcium scoring performance in cardiac computed tomography. Eur Radiol 2003; 13: 484–97

37. Hunold P, Vogt FM, Schmermund A, et al. Radiation exposure during cardiac CT: effective doses at multi-detector row CT and electron-beam CT. Radiology 2003; 226: 145–52

38. Morin RL, Gerber TC, McCollough CH. Radiation dose in computed tomography of the heart. Circulation 2003; 107: 917–22

39. Achenbach S, Giesler T, Ropers D, et al. Comparison of image quality in contrast-enhanced coronary-artery visualization by electron beam tomography and retrospectively electrocardiogram-gated multislice spiral computed tomography. Invest Radiol 2003; 38: 119–28

Calcium scoring

1. Tanenbaum SR, Kondos GT, Veselik KE, et al. Detection of calcific deposits in coronary arteries by ultrafast computed tomography and correlation with angiography. Am J Cardiol 1989; 63: 870–2

2. Agatston AS, Janowitz WR, Hildner FJ, et al. Quantification of coronary artery calcium using ultrafast computed tomography. J Am Coll Cardiol 1990; 15: 827–32

3. Breen JF, Sheedy PF 2nd, Schwartz RS, et al. Coronary artery calcification detected with ultrafast CT as an indication of coronary artery disease. Radiology 1992; 185: 435–9

4. Agatston AS, Janowitz WR, Kaplan G, et al. Ultrafast computed tomography-detected coronary calcium reflects the angiographic extent of coronary arterial atherosclerosis. Am J Cardiol 1994; 74: 1272–4

5. Mautner GC, Mautner SL, Froehlich J, et al. Coronary artery calcification: assessment with electron beam CT and histomorphometric correlation. Radiology 1994; 192: 619–23

6. Rumberger JA, Simons DB, Fitzpatrick LA, et al. Coronary artery calcium area by electron-beam computed tomography and coronary atherosclerotic plaque area. A histopathologic correlative study. Circulation 1995; 92: 2157–62

7. Wexler L, Brundage B, Crouse J, et al. Coronary artery calcification: pathophysiology, epidemiology, imaging methods, and clinical implications. A statement for health professionals from the American Heart Association. Writing Group. Circulation 1996; 94: 1175–92

8. Schmermund A, Baumgart D, Gorge G, et al. Coronary artery calcium in acute coronary syndromes: a comparative study of electron-beam computed tomography, coronary angiography, and intracoronary ultrasound in survivors of acute myocardial infarction and unstable angina. Circulation 1997; 96: 1461–9

9. Sangiorgi G, Rumberger JA, Severson A, et al. Arterial calcification and not lumen stenosis is highly correlated with atherosclerotic plaque burden in humans: a histologic study of 723 coronary artery segments using non-decalcifying methodology. J Am Coll Cardiol 1998; 89: 36–44

10. Grundy SM. Primary prevention of coronary heart disease: integrating risk assessment with intervention. Circulation 1999; 100: 988–98

11. Detrano RC, Doherty R, Wong, ND, et al. Coronary calcium does not accurately predict near-term future coronary events in high-risk adults. Circulation 1999; 99: 2633–8

12. Becker CR, Knez A, Jakobs TF, et al. Detection and quantification of coronary artery calcification with electron-beam and conventional CT. Eur Radiol 1999; 9: 620–4

13. Rumberger JA, Brundage BH, Rader DJ, Kondos G. Electron beam computed tomographic coronary calcium scanning: a review and guidelines for use in asymptomatic persons. Mayo Clin Proc 1999; 74: 243–52

14. Raggi P, Callister RQ, Cooil B. Identification of patients at increased risk of first unheralded acute myocardial infarction by electron-beam computed tomography. Circulation 2000; 101: 850–5

15. Greenland P, Abrams J, Aurigemma GP, et al. Prevention Conference V: Beyond secondary prevention: Identifying the high-risk patient for primary prevention: noninvasive tests of atherosclerotic burden: Writing Group III. Circulation 2000; 101: e16–e22

16. Jacobson TA, Griffiths GG, Varas C, et al. Impact of evidence-based 'clinical judgment' on the number of American adults requiring lipid-lowering therapy based on updated NHANES III data. National Health and Nutrition Examination Survey. Arch Intern Med 2000; 160: 1361–9

17. O'Rourke RA, Brundage BH, Froelicher VF, et al. American College of Cardiology/American Heart Association Expert Consensus document on electron-beam computed tomography for the diagnosis and prognosis of coronary artery disease. Circulation 2000; 102: 126–40

18. Smith SC Jr, Greenland P, Grundy SM. AHA Conference Proceedings. Prevention Conference V: Beyond secondary prevention: Identifying the high-risk patient for primary prevention: executive summary. American Heart Association. Circulation 2000; 101: 111–16

19. Arad Y, Spadaro LA, Goodman K, et al. Prediction of coronary events with electron beam computed tomography. J Am Coll Cardiol 2000; 36: 1253–60

20. Raggi P, Cooil B, Callister TQ. Use of electron beam tomography data to develop models for prediction of hard coronary events. Am Heart J 2001; 141: 375–82

21. Greenland P, Smith SC Jr, Grundy SM. Improving coronary heart disease risk assessment in asymptomatic people: role of traditional risk factors and noninvasive cardiovascular tests. Circulation 2001; 104: 1863–7

22. Expert Panel on Detection, Evaluation and Treatment of High Blood Cholesterol in Adults. Executive summary of the Third Report of the National Cholesterol Education Program (NCEP). J Am Med Assoc 2001; 285: 2486–97

23. Smith SC, Blair SN, Bonow RO, et al. AHA/ACC scientific statement: AHA/ACC guidelines for preventing heart attack and death in patients with atherosclerotic cardiovascular disease: 2001 update: a statement for healthcare professionals from the American Heart Association and the American College of Cardiology. Circulation 2001; 104: 1577–9

24. Haberl R, Becker A, Leber A, et al. Correlation of coronary calcification and angiographically documented stenoses in patients with suspected coronary artery dis-

ease: results of 1.764 Patients. J Am Coll Cardiol 2001; 37: 451–7

25. Schmermund A, Schwartz RS, Adamzik M, et al. Coronary atherosclerosis in unheralded sudden coronary death under age 50: histo-pathologic comparison with 'healthy' subjects dying out of hospital. Atherosclerosis 2001; 155: 499–508

26. Hoff JA, Chomka EV, Krainik AJ, et al. Age and gender distributions of coronary artery calcium detected by electron beam tomography in 35,246 adults. Am J Cardiol 2001; 87: 1335–9

27. Schmermund A, Erbel R. Unstable coronary plaque and its relation to coronary calcium. Circulation 2001; 104: 1682–7

28. Becker CR, Kleffel T, Crispin A, et al. Coronary artery calcium measurement: agreement of multirow detector and electron beam CT. Am J Roentgenol 2001; 176: 1295–8

29. Pearson TA, Blair SN, Daniels SR, et al. AHA guidelines for primary prevention of cardiovascular disease and stroke: 2002 update; consensus panel guide to comprehensive risk reduction for adult patients without coronary or other atherosclerotic vascular diseases. Circulation 2002; 106: 388–91

30. De Backer G, Ambrosioni E, Borch-Johnsen K, et al. European guidelines on cardiovascular disease prevention in clinical practice. Eur J Cardiovasc Prev Rehabil 2003; 10: s1–s10

31. Budoff MJ. Atherosclerosis imaging and calcified plaque: coronary artery disease risk assessment. Prog Cardiovasc Dis 2003; 46: 135–48

32. Hoff JA, Quinn L, Sevrukov A, et al. The prevalence of coronary artery calcium among diabetic individuals without known coronary artery disease. J Am Coll Cardiol 2003; 41: 1008–12

33. Kondos G, Hoff JA, Sevrukov A, et al. Electron-beam tomography coronary artery calcium and cardiac events. Circulation 2003; 107: 2571–6

Bypass graft and stents

1. McKay CR, Brundage BH, Ullyot DJ, et al. Evaluation of early postoperative coronary artery bypass grafts patency by contrast-enhanced computed tomography. J Am Coll Cardiol 1983; 2: 312–17

2. Barner HB, Standeven JW, Reese J. Twelve-year experience with internal mammary artery for coronary artery bypass. J Thorac Cardiovasc Surg 1985; 90: 668

3. Bateman TM, Gray RJ, Whiting JS, et al. Cine computed tomographic evaluation of aortocoronary bypass graft patency. J Am Coll Cardiol 1986; 8: 693–8

4. Bateman TM, Gray RJ, Whiting JS, et al. Prospective evaluation of ultrafast cardiac computed tomography for determination of coronary bypass graft patency. Circulation 1987; 75: 1018–24

5. Stanford W, Krachmer M, Galvin JR. Ultrafast computed tomography in assessing coronary bypass grafts. Am J Card Imaging 1991; 5: 21–8

6. Tello R, Costello P, Ecker C, Hartnell G. Spiral CT evaluation of coronary artery bypass graft patency. J Comput Assist Tomogr 1993; 17: 253–9

7. Bryan AJ, Angelini GD. The biology of saphenous vein occlusion: etiology and strategies for prevention. Curr Opin Cardiol 1994; 9: 641

8. Cameron A, Davis KB, Rogers WJ. Recurrence of angina after coronary artery bypass surgery: predictors and progression (CASS Registry). J Am Coll Cardiol 1995; 26: 895–9

9. Fitzgibbon GM, Kafka HP, Leach AJ, et al. Coronary bypass graft fate and patient outcome: angiographic follow-up of 5065 grafts related to survival and reoperation in 1388 patients during 25 years. J Am Coll Cardiol 1996; 28: 616–26

10. Schmermund A, Haude M, Baumgart D, et al. Noninvasive assessment of coronary Palmaz-Schatz stents by contrast enhanced electron beam computed tomography. Eur Heart J 1996; 17: 1546–53

11. Engelmann MG, von Smekal A, Knez A, et al. Accuracy of spiral computed tomography for identifying arterial and venous coronary graft patency. Am J Cardiol 1997; 80: 569–74

12. Achenbach S, Moshage W, Ropers D. Non-invasive, three-dimensional visualization of coronary artery bypass grafts by electron beam tomography. Am J Cardiol 1997; 79: 856–61

13. Pump H, Moehlenkamp S, Sehnert C, et al. Electron-beam CT in the noninvasive assessment of coronary stent patency. Acad Radiol 1998; 5: 858–62

14. Christenson JT, Simonet F, Schmuziger M. Sequential vein bypass grafting: tactics and long-term results. Cardiovasc Surg 1998; 6: 389–97

15. Dai R, Zhang S, Lu B, et al. Electron beam CT angiography with three-dimensional reconstruction in the evaluation of coronary artery bypass grafts. Acad Radiol 1998; 5: 863–7

16. Moehlenkamp S, Pump H, Baumgart D, et al. Minimally invasive evaluation of coronary stents with electron beam computed tomography: in vivo and in vitro experience. Catheter Cardiovasc Interv 1999; 48: 39–47

17. Ha JW, Cho SY, Shim WH, et al. Non-invasive evaluation of coronary artery bypass graft patency using three-dimensional angiography obtained with contrast-

enhanced electron beam CT. Am J Roentgenol 1999; 172: 1055–9

18. Lu B, Dai RP, Jing BL, et al. Evaluation of coronary artery bypass graft patency using three-dimensional reconstruction and flow study on electron beam tomography. J Comput Assist Tomogr 2000; 24: 663–70

19. Lu B, Dai RP, Bai H, et al. Detection and analysis of intracoronary artery stent after PTCA using contrast-enhanced three-dimensional electron beam tomography. J Invasive Cardiol 2000; 12: 1–6

20. Pump H, Moehlenkamp S, Sehnert CA, et al. Coronary arterial stent patency: assessment with electron beam CT. Radiology 2000; 214: 447–52

21. Dion R, Glineur D, Derouck D, et al. Complementary saphenous grafting: long-term follow-up. J Thorac Cardiovasc Surg 2001; 122: 296–304

22. Ropers D, Ulzheimer S, Wenkel E, et al. Investigation of aortocoronary artery bypass grafts by multislice computed tomography with electrocardiographic-gated image reconstruction. Am J Cardiol 2001; 88: 792–5

23. Nieman K, Cademartiri F, Raaijmakers R, et al. Noninvasive angiographic evaluation of coronary stents with multi-slice spiral computed tomography. Herz 2003; 28: 136–42

24. Yoo KJ, Choi D, Choi BW, et al. The comparison of the graft patency after coronary artery bypass grafting using coronary angiography and multislice computed tomography. Eur J Cardiothorac Surg 2003; 24: 86–91

25. Nieman K, Pattynama PMT, Rensing BJ, et al. CT angiographic evaluation of post-CABG patients: assessment of grafts and coronary arteries. Radiology 2003; 229: 749–56

26. Ropers D, Baum U, Anders K, et al. Contrast-enhanced multi-detector row CT with sub-millimeter collimation for the investigation of coronary artery bypass patients. Circulation 2003;(Suppl)

27. Kobuyama et al. J Am Coll Cardiol 2004; 43:A364

Coronary plaque imaging

1. Estes JM, Quist WC, Lo Gerfo FW, Costello P. Noninvasive characterization of plaque morphology using helical computed tomography. J Cardiovasc Surg (Torino) 1998; 39: 527–34

2. Becker CR, Knez A, Ohnesorge B, et al. Imaging of noncalcified coronary plaques using helical CT with retrospective ECG gating. Am J Roentgenol 2000; 175: 423–4

3. Schroeder S, Kopp AF, Baumbach A, et al. Noninvasive detection and evaluation of atherosclerotic coronary plaques with multislice computed tomography. J Am Coll Cardiol 2001; 37: 1430–5

4. Kopp AF, Schroeder S, Baumbach A, et al. Non-invasive characterisation of coronary lesion morphology and composition by multislice CT: first results in comparison with intracoronary ultrasound. Eur Radiol 2001; 11: 1607–11

5. Schroeder S, Flohr T, Kopp AF, et al. Accuracy of density measurements within plaques located in artificial coronary arteries by X-ray multislice CT: results of a phantom study. J Comput Assist Tomogr 2001; 25: 900–6

6. Schoenhagen P, Tuzcu EM, Stillman AE, et al. Non-invasive assessment of plaque morphology and remodeling in mildly stenotic coronary segments: comparison of 16-slice computed tomography and intravascular ultrasound. Coron Artery Dis 2003; 14: 459–62

7. Nikolaou K, Sagmeister S, Knez A, et al. Multidetector-row computed tomography of the coronary arteries: predictive value and quantitative assessment of non-calcified vessel-wall changes. Eur Radiol 2003; 13: 2505–12

8. Leber AW, Knez A, White CW, et al. Composition of coronary atherosclerotic plaques in patients with acute myocardial infarction and stable angina pectoris determined by contrast-enhanced multislice computed tomography. Am J Cardiol 2003; 91: 714–18

9. Caussin C, Ohanessian A, Lancelin B, et al. Coronary plaque burden detected by multislice computed tomography after acute myocardial infarction with near-normal coronary arteries by angiography. Am J Cardiol 2003; 92: 849–52

10. Becker CR, Nikolaou K, Muders M, et al. Ex vivo coronary atherosclerotic plaque characterization with multidetector-row CT. Eur Radiol 2003; 13: 2094–8

11. Achenbach S, Moselewski F, Ropers D, et al. Detection of calcified and noncalcified coronary atherosclerotic plaque by contrast-enhanced, submillimeter multidetector spiral computed tomography: a segment-based comparison with intravascular ultrasound. Circulation 2004; 109: 14–17

12. Achenbach S, Ropers D, Hoffmann U, et al. Assessment of coronary remodeling in stenotic and nonstenotic coronary atherosclerotic lesions by multidetector spiral computed tomography. J Am Coll Cardiol 2004; 43: 842–7

13. Mollet N. Non-invasive assessment of the coronary plaque burden using multi-slice computed tomography. Heart 2004 submitted

Selected reading

Blanck C, ed. Understanding Helical Scanning. Baltimore: Williams & Wilkins, 1998. ISBN 0-683-30304-X

Marcus M, Schelbert H, Skorton H, Wolf G, eds. Cardiac Imaging: A Comparison to Braunwald's Heart Disease. Part 6; Fast Computed Tomography. Philadelphia: WB Saunders, 1991:773-887. ISBN 0-7216-5862-8

Romans LE, ed. Introduction to Computed Tomography. Baltimore: Williams &Wilkins,1995. ISBN 0-683-07353-2

Seeram E, ed. Computed Tomography: Physical Principles, Clinical Applications and Quality Control. Philadelphia: WB Saunders, 2001. ISBN 0721681735

Index